# ENIGMAS of HEALTH and DISEASE

Also by Alfredo Morabia

*Epidémiologie causale: Principes, Exemples, Théorie*
(Geneva: Médecine et Hygiène, 1996)
*L'épidémiologie clinique: Que-Sais-je?*
(Paris: Presse Universitaires de France, 1996)
*L'epidemiologia clinica*
(Rome: Il Pensiero Scientifico Editore, 1999)
*History of Epidemiologic Methods and Concepts*
(Basel, Birkhauser, 2004)
*Le Bus Santé: une aventure genevoise*
(Geneva: Médecine et Hygiène, 2006)
*Psychiatric Epidemiology: Searching for the Causes of Mental Disorders* (with E. Susser, S. Schwartz, and E. Bromet)
(Oxford: Oxford University Press, 2006)

ALFREDO MORABIA

# ENIGMAS

OF

# HEALTH

AND

# DISEASE

HOW EPIDEMIOLOGY HELPS
UNRAVEL SCIENTIFIC MYSTERIES

COLUMBIA UNIVERSITY PRESS

NEW YORK

Columbia University Press
*Publishers Since 1893*
New York    Chichester, West Sussex
cup.columbia.edu

Adapted from *Santé: Distinguer croyances et connaissance*
Copyright © 2011 ODILE JACOB, Paris / Pr Alfredo Morabia
Translation Copyright © 2014 Columbia University Press

Library of Congress Cataloging-in-Publication Data

Morabia, Alfredo, author.
Enigmas of health and disease : how epidemiology helps unravel scientific
mysteries / Alfredo Morabia.
p. ; cm.
Adaptation of: *Santé* / Alfredo Morabia. 2011.
Includes bibliographical references and index.
ISBN 978-0-231-16884-7 (cloth : alk. paper) — ISBN 978-0-231-16885-4
(pbk. : alk. paper —ISBN 978-0-231-53767-4 (ebook)
I. Morabia, Alfredo, *Santé*. Adaptation of (work) : II. Title.
[DNLM: 1. Epidemiology. WA 105]
RA652
614.4—dc23
2013046811

Columbia University Press books are printed on permanent
and durable acid-free paper.
This book is printed on paper with recycled content.
Printed in the United States of America
c 10 9 8 7 6 5 4 3 2 1
p 10 9 8 7 6 5 4 3 2

Cover design: Faceout Studio, Tim Green
Cover image: General Research Division, The New York Public Library,
Astor, Lenox and Tilden Foundations

References to websites (URLs) were accurate at the time of writing.
Neither the author nor Columbia University Press is responsible for URLs
that may have expired or changed since the manuscript was prepared.

To Léon and Bob

# CONTENTS

# PREFACE TO THE ENGLISH EDITION

THE BOOK you are reading is the English *adaptation* of my 2011 French book entitled *Santé: Distinguer croyances et connaissance.* My original approach to translating *Santé* had been to remain faithful to its words, style, and syntax. This proved ineffective, however, because it ignored a key component of language: the cultural context. While I am writing now, each word comes to my mind with a choice of synonyms, reminiscent of books, songs, or poems. In both French and English, words, expressions, and syntax flexibility are nested in different sets of cultural and literary connections. On top of this, English-speaking societies are more familiar with epidemiology than French-speaking ones and therefore necessitate different narration.

My last incentive to adapt rather than translate *Santé* is more personal. I had grown tired of reading the same prose in both English and French and yearned to feel the same excitement from the English version I had from the book in French. The result is that although *Santé* and *Enigmas of Health and Disease* cover the same topics and develop the same ideas, each book has its own distinct character.

I made two notable changes. Following the recommendations of my reviewers and American publisher, I dropped a chapter highlighting the use of epidemiology in everyday life when one is reading newspapers, magazine, and blogs. Although relevant, it detracted from the main thread: the historical process by which society embraced epidemiology to unravel scientific mysteries. Instead, I added a new section describing the complexity of distinguishing a variety of possible causes to a health event.

This differs from my original intention to expose each enigma as if it involved only a single cause (e.g., physical activity) and a single outcome. (e.g., breast cancer) The new section allowed me to offer a more accurate representation of epidemiologists and their permanent concern with discerning causality. Now this concern is discussed in chapter 14, "Group Comparisons Also Fail."

A section, unfortunately absent in *Santé*, describes the fascinating study about the causes of breast cancer conducted in 1926 by Janet Lane-Claypon. Lane-Claypon is an important female epidemiologist who contributed to the evolution of the methods for comparing groups before World War II. Her contribution was original and substantial.[1]

My books grow out of my teaching. I am therefore grateful to all the students across the world who have attended my lectures, listened critically, and made constructive comments and suggestions as well as to Albert Hofman, Ezra Susser, Sandro Galea, Moyses Szklo, Michelle Williams, and the late Patricia Buffler, who have been instrumental, in some way or another, in allowing me to work on these ideas and teach them. I have received comments on the whole or parts of the manuscript (French or English) from (in alphabetic order) Michael C. Costanza, Randi Epstein, Dan Fox, Steven Goodman, Miguel Hernan, Serge Hercberg, Bob Morabia, Herman van Oyen, Arthur L. Rheingold, Jonathan Samet, Alan Sipress, Linda Stroun, Ulrich Troehler, and Jan P. Vandenbroucke. I have benefited from discussions over the years with the editors of the James Lind Library (www.jameslindlibrary.org), Jan P. Vandenbroucke, Ulrich Troehler, Iain Milne, Iain Chalmers, the historians Anne Hardy and Iain Donaldson, and my friends and colleagues Steven Markowitz, Miquel Porta, Steve Stellman, Shiriki Kumnayika, Sonia Hernandez-Diaz, Sander Greenland, Sharon Schwartz, Mary Wolff, David Rosner, Cesar Victora, Raj Bohpal, Roger Bernier, Gerald Oppenheimer, and Alex Broadbent. It would be unfair not to acknowledge, besides these intellectual inputs, the coaches of Team New York Aquatics for the biweekly workouts and the folks from New York City Swim for the open-water swims around Manhattan and their commitment to "taking back the rivers." They are my psychotropic agents. Léon Morabia, senior student at Wheaton College, Massachusetts, serves as my communications strategist and currently manages my social media and online presence. The People's Epidemiology Library (www. epidemiology.ch/history/PeopleEpidemiologyLibrary.html), which Jan Vandenbroucke and I edit, provides many of the historical references cited in this book. Zoey Laskaris, who assists my epidemiological and historical research, proved to be a gifted editor, both for style and content. On the bibliographic side, I was helped by the talented librarian Charles R. Fikar and the librarians at the Columbia University Health Science Library.

It has been a pleasure to collaborate with Patrick Fitzgerald from Columbia University Press and Marie Morvan from Odile Jacob Publisher, who made this English adaptation possible. Bridget Flannery-McCoy and Kathryn Schell prepared the manuscript for publication. Annie Barva polished the final version for style, syntax, and consistency. Daniel Fox did me the grand favor of meticulously reading the proofs to eliminate the last traces of too literal, French translations.

The only source of funding that had some relevance for the preparation of this book is a grant from the National Library of Medicine (1G13LM010884).

# PROLOGUE

## A Science Named Epidemiology

WHETHER YOU are consumer of health services, practicing clinician, health professional in training, health journalist, epidemiologist, or epidemiology student, this book explains how and why epidemiology has evolved in 350 years from being a science of epidemics to being indispensable for the discovery of effective ways of preventing health harms, prolonging life, and treating diseases.

To solve enigmas of health and diseases, epidemiology has become a science that compares groups of people. Group comparisons are a tool to study the health effects of many aspects of human life, including lifestyle factors such as tobacco smoking, lack of exercise, excess caloric intake, oral contraceptive use, alcohol; social conditions such as education, income, occupation, and neighborhood; and environmental exposure such as air pollution. Comparing groups is also at the core of the scientific methods needed to assess the efficacy of medical procedures for prevention and treatment.

Here is an example of group comparison: take a group of people who exercise and another who don't. For the following ten years, count all the new cases of heart attacks occurring in each of the groups. At the end of the ten years, compare the frequency of heart attacks in each of the two groups. If exercise protects, you would expect heart attacks to be less frequent among the active than among the inactive group. Thus, in its simplest form, a group comparison can be used to determine whether a disease occurs more often in a group that is exposed to some factor than in a group that is not exposed to that factor.

Most of the time, performing a group comparison is the only option to identify causes of diseases or whether treatments work. Think of all you know about the health effects of tobacco, diet, physical activity, occupational exposures, screening tests, drugs, medical care, social and economic living conditions, and other aspects of your life that may impact your health. Think of questions such as: What is a healthy diet? How many times per week should we exercise? Is this drug effective? Should we put babies to sleep on their belly or on their back? And so on for the health effects of sunscreen, alcohol, tobacco, drugs, contraception, and safe sex. If some scientific knowledge exists about the health consequences of these issues, it most likely is a find based on group comparisons.

I use the term *knowledge* as opposed to *beliefs*. Don't read it as a synonym of truth, but rather of evidence. I prefer to speak of knowledge than of evidence. Group comparisons produce data. These data are tangible; they can be evaluated, criticized, and then confirmed, or not. Whether the results of a group comparison are confirmed or not, whether they were true or untrue, we have learned something, we are more knowledgeable and can progress. We have the option of getting more data, better data, different data to improve our knowledge. In contrast, beliefs are products of our imagination. They are mere opinions with which we can agree or disagree, but whose origin we cannot evaluate. When I say cigarettes don't cause cancer because my neighbor who is now ninety-five has smoked since he was fifteen and does not have any cancer, I express my belief based on my interpretation of a selected observation. You may be of a different opinion because a good friend of yours, a smoker, died at age fifty of lung cancer. We may argue forever, no one being able to tell who is right or who is wrong until we can rely on knowledge. This example may seem mundane, but many, many circulating health statements on important issues, such as vaccines, are of that sort.

I am not saying that we should discard opinions and beliefs. As the nineteenth-century German professor of hygiene Max von Pettenkofer used to say, "If we had to live only on what has been ascertained scientifically, all of us, as many as we are, would have perished long ago."[1] We need health beliefs. They are part of us and cannot be dissociated from us. My point is that it is important to distinguish knowledge from belief.

Group comparisons can help us do that with regard to health issues. Most of the health claims we find on the Internet or among our acquaintances are beliefs. Considering these beliefs on a par with knowledge can be a source of unwarranted anxiety or of ill decisions. My claim in this book is very simple and unpretentious: checking whether a health statement is based on a group comparison or not is an effective way of separating health knowledge from health belief.

Epidemiology is already important in our everyday life. Where does the knowledge supporting the warnings on packs of cigarettes about the dangers of tobacco come from? Epidemiology. Why do you trust that the screening test recommended by your doctor can contribute to your living longer? Epidemiology. Which science provides the methods to determine whether surgery is effective for lower back pain? Epidemiology. In 2009, David Leonhardt asked Barack Obama "how going to the doctor will be different in the future; how they will experience medical care differently on the other side of health-care reform." In his answer, the president emphasized "the importance of using comparative-effectiveness studies as a way of reining in costs" and the possibility for doctors to say to patients: "You know what, we've looked at some objective studies out here, people who know about this stuff, concluding that the blue pill, which costs half as much as the red pill, is just as effective, and you might want to go ahead and get the blue one."[2] What are the "comparative-effectiveness studies" that President Obama mentioned in relation to the health-care reform? Epidemiology.

Thus, epidemiology is the science underlying most of the practical knowledge about whether measures to prevent and treat illness work. There is, of course, a wealth of other health knowledge that is not based on epidemiology, related to the anatomy, physiology, and pathology of the human body; to the cellular effects of drugs or microorganisms; to the molecular structure of the toxicological and infectious causes of diseases; and so on. The full list of all the domains in which health knowledge progresses without resorting to group comparisons would be very long. But rarely do they provide knowledge that is immediately relevant for prevention, treatment, or screening.

## EPIDEMIOLOGY IN THE MEDIA

The results of group comparisons can be found daily in the health sections of newspapers and magazines. Here are some titles gleaned from English-speaking media:

"Walking Six Miles Each Week Could Reduce Chance of Getting Alzheimer's" (*Daily Mail*, United Kingdom, November 29, 2010)[3]

"Cell Phones and Cancer: A Study's Muddled Findings" (*Time*, May 17, 2010)[4]

"People Who Drink as Few as Two Soft Drinks a Week Face Nearly Twice the Risk of Developing Deadly Cancer, Study Finds" (*CBSNews Healthwatch*, February 9, 2010)

"Diet: Eating Fish Found to Ward Off Eye Disease" (*New York Times*, March 22, 2011)

"Scientists Identify Genes for 'Extreme Longevity'" (*AOL News*, July 1, 2010)

"Alzheimer's Gene 'Linked to Vitamin D'" (*Telegraph*, May 30, 2011)

"Politicians Should Not Prescribe Pills" (*Financial Time*, July 14, 2010)

"Progestin: Hormone Replacement Therapy Study Halted" (*CNN Health*, July 9, 2002)

"Good Week for People Who Make Their Grievances Heard at Work" (*The Australian*, May 28, 2011)

"Vitamins 'Lower Risk of Autism'" (*Sydney Morning Herald*, May 27, 2011)

"Research Shows Extra Calcium Unnecessary" (*The West Australian*, May 25, 2011)

"Study Shows Caffeine Might Prevent Pregnancy" (*Ottawa Citizen*, May 25, 2011)[5]

All of these articles comment on the results of group comparisons performed using epidemiologic methods. Some news agencies have specific epidemiology sections on their websites, reporting the results of group comparisons.[6]

Even though epidemiology's importance has grown in our everyday life, I suspect many people do not recognize it every time they come across its results. Several explanations come to mind for this relative lack of visibility.

## EPIDEMIO-LOGY

Most medical specialties are named according to their subject matter: cardiology deals with the heart, gastroenterology with the stomach and the gut, neurology with the nervous system, and so on. The same is true for most human and social sciences, such as sociology, psychology, economics. What is epidemiology about?

When I introduce myself as an epidemiologist, people sometimes seek advice for a skin problem because they think I am an "epidermologist." More often they will ask: "Oh, you must be knowledgeable about the HIV epidemic?" To which I reply, "Not particularly, sorry."

The fact is that equating epidemiology with the science of epidemics is etymologically correct. The term *epidemiology* literarily evokes a medical specialty that deals with contagious epidemics. Indeed, in the nineteenth century epidemiology was the science of epidemics. The recurrent epidemics of cholera, a scourge that periodically ravaged the world, stimulated the creation of a professional association of epidemiologists in 1850 called the London Epidemiologic Society.[7]

Today's epidemiology, however, does not exclusively study infectious diseases. Its scope has expanded to the identification of all determinants of human health, whether they occur as epidemics, with rapidly changing frequencies over short periods of time, or not. Epidemiology is apt to study the health effects of many characteristics of human life. It also provides the science needed to assess whether medical procedures, treatments, and screening tests are salutary.

The examples used in this book and the headlines mentioned earlier give an idea of the breadth of topics to which epidemiology can be applied in order to assist in the acquisition of health knowledge.

## METHODS VERSUS MATTER

Why did epidemiology keep its nineteenth-century name if it no longer applies? Maybe because it is challenging to give a name to a mode of research characterized by the use of group comparisons. Epidemiology is not associated with a particular domain of medicine or public health.

All domains of medicine and public health rely on epidemiology. In the "war" against cancer, the "battle" against polio, the "fight" against obesity and alcoholism, or the "struggle" against health inequalities, epidemiology provides the strategists, not the domain experts. Experts are, respectively, cancerologists, vaccinologists, nutritionists, alcohologists, and social scientists. Some experts may also be epidemiologists, and epidemiologists may also be domain experts, but the strictly epidemiologic component of the endeavor is to identify the populations to be compared and the modes of collecting, organizing, and interpreting the data.

The crucial role of epidemiology can elude the public because its methodologic contribution remains in the background when the results of a study are disseminated. The discovery of an anticholesterol drug that decreases the risk of heart attacks appears as a success of cardiology or lipidology rather than of epidemiology even though the design and conduct of the study relied on epidemiology.

## SCIENCE AND KNOW-HOW

Because epidemiology has an ambiguous name and an activity often out of public view, its contribution to health knowledge is not always obvious. On top of these obstacles we add its theoretical complexity. Comparing groups requires a scientific training and a know-how that pertain to epidemiologists. Are experts really needed to identify comparable groups? The answer is yes. Epidemiologists are experts at identifying and recruiting groups of people that can reasonably be compared. This is not a trivial activity.

Some group comparisons have simpler designs than others. For example, there are experimental designs in which a potentially beneficial treatment is attributed to some patients but not to others using a chance procedure equivalent to tossing a coin. In such randomized controlled trials (a term explained in chapter 8), it is easy to perceive that the groups will be comparable. A great deal of the difficulty is technical and lies in the performance of the experiment. These trials are ideal for evaluating whether treatments have beneficial health effects or not. At the same time, it is not possible to toss a coin to allocate a potentially deleterious exposure or behavior. Would you prescribe either a pack of cigarettes containing true tobacco or cigarettes free of tar and nicotine to (up to then) nonsmokers in order to determine if the health of those who smoke true tobacco declines faster than of those who smoke fake tobacco? Of course not, and therefore the effects of tobacco products on health need to be studied with people who have already chosen to smoke or not. Both groups differ substantially beyond their smoking habits. They live different lives and have different motivations for participating in epidemiologic studies. How can we reach out to them? How can we ensure that the findings among people who agree to participate in the study are relevant for the population at large? These situations cry for creative study designs; otherwise, the results will be fraught with error and invalid.

Let me use here an example from my own experience. My colleagues and I conducted one of the first group comparisons of whether women who smoke cigarettes or who breathe air polluted by cigarette smokers were at increased breast cancer risk.[8] Jane Brody of the *New York Times* asked, "Could cigarette smoking account for the mysteriously rising incidence of breast cancer among American women?" She went on to describe the design of the group comparison: "The study, conducted among 244 women with breast cancer and 1,032 women free of the disease, revealed that the more a woman smoked, the greater were her chances of having breast cancer. Thus, for women who smoked less than half a pack a day, the breast cancer risk was doubled; for those who smoked 10 to 19 cigarettes a day, the risk was 2.7 times greater, and for those who smoked a pack or more a day, the risk was 4.6 times greater."[9]

In that study, we carefully tried to recruit all new cases of breast cancer in the population over a two-year period. We simultaneously drew a random sample of the general population to serve as comparison group. We interviewed the participants about their lifelong exposure to active and passive smoking. The fact that smoking was more common in women diagnosed with breast cancer than among comparable women who weren't did not necessarily imply that smoking caused breast cancer. Because breast cancer is more common in women who never had children, we needed to make sure that this was not the reason for the observed difference. If nonsmokers have more children, then that might be the explanation behind their lower risk of breast cancer. The same reasoning applied for all the known and postulated causes of breast cancer. There are alternative explanations and methodological errors to consider before presenting an observed relation as potentially causal.

The conduct of group comparisons requires a theoretical background taught in schools of public health[10] and a technical know-how acquired through practice. This book is not about epidemiologists' theoretical background or know-how.

## THIS IS NOT A TEXTBOOK

The book you are reading is not a "popular" textbook of epidemiology because no technical expertise in these methods is required to use epidemiology in everyday life. When epidemiologic results become accessible to the public in newspapers, in popular media, or on the Internet, they usually have already been deemed valuable by the scientific community. Their authors have, in principle, already convinced the scientific journal editors and experts that their findings were rigorous enough to be published and shared with others. At that stage, when results become news for the public, the technical aspects of the group comparison are not crucial anymore. Readers of public news media need to be able to understand how the groups were compared, who was compared, and how much health benefit or health harm was observed. This book addresses the public's need.

Even knowledge of math is unnecessary. Of course, epidemiologists use statistical techniques to analyze the data they collect. These methods can be quite sophisticated, but the users of a statistical analysis do not need to understand the mechanics of that analysis to be able to interpret the study results. The statistical component of epidemiologic studies is rarely if ever mentioned in the news coverage of epidemiologic findings. It is extremely unusual for a newspaper to mention whether "the number of participants was large enough to detect the effect of a treatment or of a preventive factor if it existed" or to provide "the probability that similar or more extreme findings would have been observed in another study if there were no association." Epidemiologic and statistical expertise is needed before the results are disseminated. It is not crucial after that point. I hope to convince you of that.

However, the concepts explained in my book, such as population thinking and group comparisons, are noble. I did not try to vulgarize them or simplify them in order to make them accessible, as I would have had to do for statistical or technical issues. What you can learn in this book about epidemiology you will not have to learn again or in a different way. But if your interest in epidemiology has been piqued by this book, I recommend that you consult a more traditional text that presents the basic concepts and methods.

Overall, epidemiology's great contribution to health care and public health lies in a fairly simple discovery: group comparisons are indispensable to acquire health knowledge about prevention, treatment, and screening efficacy. Because this truth does not make intuitive sense, it took several centuries and many enigmas of health and disease to become commonly accepted. It is the historical sequence of some of the scientific mysteries epidemiology unraveled that I will replay in the coming chapters.

## TIMELINE

For those who wonder how to approach the chapters of this book, here is some information that may be useful. First, regarding the order in which the chapters can be read. Each chapter stands alone, but there is a timeline across chapters 2 to 13. Chapter 2 goes until the end of the sixteenth century; chapter 3 covers the seventeenth and eighteenth centuries; chapters 4 and 5 cover the nineteenth century; chapter 6 covers the first half of the twentieth century; chapter 7 covers the second half of the twentieth century; and chapters 8 to 13 are about the end of the twentieth and beginning of the twenty-first centuries.

In order to avoid technical digressions in the main text, I have added four appendixes, written in the same style as the rest of the book, for readers who want to follow the technical discussion in more detail.

Finally, the notes link the text to the bibliography and allow you to find the sources or explore a topic further. In the notes, articles and books are cited by the author's name followed by the year of publication (e.g., Snow 1855) because the full reference can be found in the bibliography.

## CONFLICT OF INTEREST

People who read the French edition of this book have asked me where the financial resources to write and publish it came from. Did some industry support me? Could some of my statements be tainted by the need to protect my sponsors' interests? I found these questions absolutely legitimate. After all, I used to ask every person who published in *Preventive Medicine*, the journal I was chief editor of, to sign a conflict-of-interest form disclosing any link to corporate interests, which might alter the researcher's independence. Why would I not be similarly obligated to my readers?

This disclosure is quite simple. I did not receive support from corporate sources. I used the material and documents from the lectures I give in various academic settings and wrote the book mostly during my spare time. A 2012 three-year grant from the US National Library of Medicine has allowed me to dedicate much more time to study the history of epidemiology. Even though the National Library of Medicine project is not directly related to this English adaptation of *Santé*, it has definitely increased my expertise in the topics covered in this book. My publishers, Odile Jacob in France and Columbia University Press in the United States, have been responsible for the cost of publication of this book.

# ENIGMAS of HEALTH and DISEASE

# 1

## COMPARING GROUPS AND
## THE FIFTH DIMENSION

CONSIDER THIS health claim from *Glamour* magazine: "Great health news for every woman. Quick! Take this poll: If there were a pill that could . . . 'Slash your chances of getting breast cancer / Help get rid of headaches / Cut symptoms of depression almost in half / Lower your risk of type 2 diabetes by 50 percent / Make it easier to get pregnant when you want to / Boost sexual arousal by 100 percent / Improve your body image / Make you fall asleep 40 percent faster / And help you lose up to a pound a week' . . . Would you take it? Who wouldn't? Well, here's the deal: There is no new miracle pill, but research showing that you can get all these benefits from 30 minutes of daily exercise keeps piling up. (The latest study finds that regular workouts can reduce your risk of memory problems by a third.)"[1]

If the article tells the truth, how do we know that, to take the first claimed benefit, "30 minutes of daily exercise slash the chances of getting breast cancer"? The answer cannot be found peeping through a microscope or putting mice on a treadmill. Studying the occurrence of breast cancer among physically active women would not suffice either because we would not know how often breast cancer would have been diagnosed had these women engaged in less physical activity. The only way to know whether "30 minutes of daily exercise slash the risk of getting breast cancer" is to compare groups of women. If there is objective evidence underlying all the benefits of regular workouts claimed by *Glamour*, it must come from group comparisons. Epidemiology must have provided the methods to compare physically active and sedentary women to know whether one of the two groups is at greater risk of breast cancer than the other or to compare women diagnosed with breast cancer and women free of breast cancer to determine if one of the two groups used to be more active than the other.

In this sense, *Glamour*'s statement about the multifarious benefits of physical activity is missing key information needed to interpret it. Can you tell what groups were compared? One group of women did at least thirty minutes of daily exercise, but what about the women in the comparison group? Did they do less than thirty minutes of daily physical activity or no physical activity at all? This is a crucial bit of information. I would also like to know how much risk reduction is meant by "slash." Without this information, the implication of the statement for a woman's life remains vague.

## COMPARING GROUPS

Figure 1.1 depicts the information I would like to find in an article reporting the results of a group comparison to the general public. I use the same format to illustrate graphically the results of other group comparisons described in this book. Data come from a French study[2] conducted among female teachers.

Each bar of figure 1.1 represents a group. Duration of physical activity is on the horizontal axis and breast cancer risk is on the vertical axis. The left bar indicates that five hours or more of vigorous physical activity is associated with an annual risk of breast cancer of 24.4 per 10,000 women or 0.24 percent per year.[3] The right bar indicates the risk of the sedentary women: 38.1 per 10,000 women per year, or 0.38 percent per year.

These tiny annual risks most likely do not mean much for you. However, cumulated over thirty years, they add up to 7.3 percent among the active women and 11.4 percent among the sedentary women, which is more meaningful.[4]

Whether we consider the annual risks or the thirty-year risks, in this population the risk of women performing at least five hours of vigorous physical activity per week is "slashed" compared to that of the women who do none.

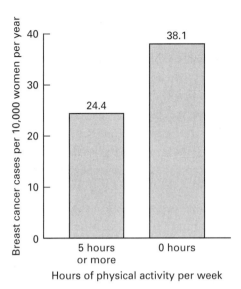

FIGURE 1.1  **Breast Cancer Rate in France, 1990–2002**

Annual risks of breast cancer among healthy French women ages forty to sixty-five followed up between 1990 and 2002, according to the weekly amount of vigorous physical activity. Risk is 24.4 per year per 10,000 women performing five hours or more of vigorous physical activity per week and 38.1 per year per 10,000 women who do not engage in vigorous physical activity at all.

*Source*: Tehard et al. 2006.

This is what the data show. Did this additional information modify your interpretation of the message in the article from *Glamour* quoted earlier? Personally, I note that the reported benefit is computed relative to the complete absence of physical activity during leisure time. Benefit will be less important for women who already do between zero and five hours of vigorous physical activity weekly. And I am impressed by the magnitude of the benefit. A breast cancer risk reduction of several percentage points for women who would switch from no activity to at least forty minutes per day of vigorous physical activity for thirty years is considerable.

I usually will not base my opinion on the results of a single study. I would like to know if other group comparisons have found similar results and if there is a biological mechanism explaining such a large risk reduction. But I will keep these results in mind until I eventually become convinced or dissuaded that the claim can be taken seriously.

You can argue that at the end my take of these results remains a question of belief, whether it is based on epidemiologic data or on other sources. There is a major difference, however. If I am under the impression that physical activity does not protect against breast cancer because I have known physically active women who nevertheless developed breast cancer, my personal opinion cannot be generalized. You may have a different opinion, and there is no way we can tell if one of us is right.

In contrast, the evidence presented in figure 1.1 can be evaluated and criticized. We can compare it with the results of similar studies, scrutinize their methodology, and search for an explanatory mechanism through which physical activity may reduce risk. Whether one agrees with the evidence or not, it provides an objective basis upon which a critical discussion can take place. In that sense, the evidence in figure 1.1 contributes to our knowledge about how to reduce the risk of breast cancer even when it still needs to be confirmed or contradicted by additional evidence.

Actually, the answer to the simple question "Is this health claim based on a group comparison?" is the first step to separating beliefs from knowledge.

Consider now other health news found in an article about natural therapy titled "Cooling Cucumbers," which announces that cooled slices of cucumber are a "tried and trusted remedy used by generations of women to reduce under-eye bags." "Cucumber slices stored in the fridge and applied to the eyes will help to soothe puffy eyes." "Lay slices on your eyes and relax for ten minutes or so. The eye area should feel refreshed and plumped."[5]

How do we know that cucumber slices help to soothe puffy eyes? The information provided does not allow us to answer the question. Was the application of cucumber slices compared to the application of humid, cucumber-free compresses for the same duration in a sufficient number of people? These are important questions to clarify. If the treatment works, why not use it? But in the absence of a group comparison, we cannot determine if it is based on knowledge or belief.

# DOES ASPIRIN PROTECT AGAINST
# HEART ATTACKS?

You may argue that one does not need to use a group comparison to know whether aspirin calms pain. If I have pain, I know the aspirin will relieve it. Why bother?

Yes, some treatments have spectacular effects. The pain-reducing effect of aspirin is a no-brainer. It has been known for thousands of years. Native American Indians and Hottentot shepherds of South Africa used to calm pain with infusion of the bark of willow trees—which contains salicylic acid, the active ingredient of aspirin—long before the synthesis of aspirin.[6] The story is worth telling.

On April 14, 1876, Frederick Ensor, a British medical doctor practicing in South Africa, sent an open letter to the editor of *The Lancet*, a prestigious English medical journal. Ensor reacted to a recent publication in this leading medical journal about the efficacy of aspirin in the treatment of rheumatoid arthritis, a chronic, inflammatory disease of the joints. His letter described the case of a South African patient suffering from a severe crisis of rheumatoid arthritis, which he tried to treat unsuccessfully using mercury, but who was cured when "[an] old Hottentot shepherd had made her a decoction of the shoots of the willows which grow on the banks of the river."[7] The Hottentot shepherd used a natural form of aspirin, whereas the medical doctor applied a treatment based on a wrong theory of disease causation. The Hottentot had been able to discover an effective treatment by trial and error because of the spectacular analgesic effect of salicylic acid. In contrast, Ensor would have needed a group comparison to determine whether mercury ever worked.

But is the effect of aspirin on the heart a no-brainer, too? Forty years ago some astute practitioners observed that patients admitted for heart attacks in a Boston hospital consumed less aspirin than similar patients admitted for diagnoses other than heart attack.[8] Also, in laboratory experiments aspirin prevented blood coagulation. Was there a link between these two observations? Could the anticoagulant effect of aspirin protect against heart attacks? The hypothesis was plausible. Heart attacks can be caused by the formation of clots in the coronary arteries that irrigate the heart muscle. Logically, a drug that prevents the formation of these clots should also prevent heart attack. But this is only a belief as long as it is not confirmed by a group comparison.

We would not know today that aspirin protects against heart attacks without the group comparisons conducted among people differing in their aspirin consumption. Several scientists compared one group receiving aspirin (at daily doses varying from 75 milligrams for a "baby aspirin" to 500 milligrams for a regular-strength aspirin) with another receiving a dummy pill, called a placebo, that looked like aspirin but did not contain salicylic acid. A chance procedure, equivalent to the toss of a fair coin, was used to decide who would receive the baby aspirin and who the placebo. Participants took either the aspirin or the placebo daily for several months, during which new cases of heart attacks were counted.

How much health benefit was observed? These studies collectively show that 500 milligrams or less of aspirin per day reduces the rate of coronary artery disease from 52 per 10,000 per year to 37 per 10,000 per year.[9] These rates do not mean much for an individual. Their difference (52 − 37 = 15) indicates that fifteen heart attacks will be prevented for 10,000 people who take aspirin daily for a year. This is still not very intuitive, but try this: if 10,000 prescriptions are needed to prevent fifteen heart attacks, how many prescriptions are needed to prevent one heart attack? A simple cross-multiplication will give you the answer.[10]

Did you find that 667 people taking aspirin for one year are needed to prevent one heart attack? The 666 other people will have no personal benefit. Clearly, taking the aspirin and observing its effects in our body will not suffice to perceive the protective effect of aspirin against heart attacks. Doubting its protective effect is more likely. Imagine asking these 667 people for their opinion! The reality is that most treatments, preventive factors, and screening programs have an effect magnitude closer to the inconspicuous cardioprotection conferred by aspirin than to its dramatic analgesic properties. The expression "No group comparison, no health knowledge" is the rule rather than the exception.

## THE FIFTH DIMENSION

Do you recall the message that said, "Cucumber slices stored in the fridge and applied to the eyes will help to soothe puffy eyes"? The message is easier to understand than the relation between physical activity and breast cancer because it pretends that satisfaction is guaranteed. Apply the cucumber slices, and your puffy eyes should feel rested! In contrast, the epidemiological study on breast cancer does not say: "Exercise vigorously five hours weekly, and you will not have breast cancer." Although the absence of this conclusion is frustrating, the reason behind it is quite simple: the question asked by the individual ("Will exercise free me from having breast cancer?") and the question addressed by the group comparison ("Does exercise prevent breast cancer?") are different.

There is no answer to the question "Will exercise free me from having breast cancer?" If a particular woman exercised five hours daily over thirty years and did not get breast cancer, we will never know if exercise played a role in the latter.

However, a group comparison can address the question "Does exercise prevent breast cancer?" The answer is a tentative "yes" if breast cancer is less frequent among active women than among sedentary women. Women who engage in regular exercise place themselves in a subgroup of the population with a lower risk of developing breast cancer.

The results shown in figure 1.1 serve to indicate to women ages forty to sixty-five years that engaging in regular exercise places them in the group on the left, at lower risk of developing breast cancer, whereas being sedentary places them in the group on the right, at higher risk of breast cancer. It is however impossible to predict which twenty four individuals out of 10,000 active women, or which 38 individuals out of 10,000 sedentary women will develop breast cancer each year. There is nothing complicated here once we understand the proper interpretation of the results of group comparisons. Nevertheless, transitioning from an individual form of thinking ("Will it work for me?") to a population form of thinking ("Does it work?") is an obstacle everyone encounters when approaching epidemiology. We are not used to this transition. We are not prepared for "population thinking" by our physiological intellectual development. We don't spontaneously think in terms of populations and risks.

Because thinking based on populations is so different from our usual individual form of thinking, I have come to view it as a fifth dimension, beyond space and time. Moving up and down, left or right, forward and backward is commonsensical. Time may be difficult to explain but we feel its clockwise flight. However, many enigmas of health and disease can be solved only in an intelligible but not sensible universe inhabited by populations. Thus, nimbly moving from our perceptible world, dominated by individuals and chance, to a universe in which we are unidentifiable members of larger but predictable groups of people is a skill we need to learn. In chapter 15, I propose one way of teaching this skill to students.

## SEPARATING KNOWLEDGE FROM BELIEF

Using epidemiology to separate knowledge from belief can be beneficial to our individual health, but it is also crucial for our collective health. Epidemiology is indispensable for decision making in public health. Let us consider a recent example of very broad relevance in which there has been a vivid tension between beliefs and knowledge: the epidemic of swine flu and its H1N1 virus.

Remember when in the spring of 2009 a new influenza virus that originally infected pork began to infect humans and spread rapidly across the world. The new virus was of the same type as that of the Great Influenza Epidemic of 1918, which killed millions of mostly young adults all over the planet. If the new virus was as dangerous as its 1918 ancestor, public-health authorities had the responsibility to prevent its potentially dreadful consequences.

Unlike in 1918, today we have a tool against the flu: vaccines. Because the body's ability to generate an immune response (antibodies) for the flu virus does not provide long-term protection as do vaccine against other disease agents, such as diphtheria, tetanus, pertussis, and so on, flu vaccines are not as effective as the standard vaccines recommended for every child. Vaccinologists have developed strategies to take this instability into account, but a vaccine providing adequate immunity can sometimes be prepared only at the last minute. It is a race against time to protect vaccinees against a severe flu. Vaccinations are expected to slow the progression of the epidemic, prevent deaths, and avoid overcrowding of health services. In the case of the H1N1 virus, commonly referred to as "swine flu," the process of selecting the new flu strain and making the vaccine was more or less identical to the annual process of strain selection and vaccine production for the seasonal flu. The only difference was that all this had to be done in a shorter period of time, starting in April or so instead of the usual February.

In the summer of 2009, most public-health authorities around the world agreed that vaccinating the entire population would maximize the chances of avoiding a possible ordeal. As a result, they marshaled their industries and health services to do so.

In the United States, the objective was to vaccinate "as many people as possible . . . as quickly as possible." The initial target group for vaccination comprised pregnant women, people who live with or care for infants younger than six months of age, and health-care and emergency medical services personnel. The government bought 229 million doses of H1N1 vaccine.[11] But the public did not follow this lead. Among all persons age six months or older, 2009 H1N1 vaccination coverage nationally was 27.0 percent.[12]

Was it wrong to plan a systematic vaccination of the whole US population in 2009 to face the threat of the H1N1 epidemic? Here are the terms of the problem that public-health authorities were facing.

The virus was potentially devastating, particularly for children. At the same time, a vaccine with similar immunogenicity and safety as seasonal vaccines could be prepared. This was a viable option because public-health authorities knew that the seasonal flu vaccine was safe. Its safety had been tested using comparative studies in which groups of people who received the vaccine were compared with groups of similar people who did not receive it. These group comparisons showed that vaccinated people developed antibodies against the flu virus and that the adverse effects of the vaccine are mostly mild, such as pain at the injection site or low fever or muscle aches. Substances called "adjuvant" increasing the body's immune response to the vaccine and thus sparing antigen—not used in the United States for the H1N1 vaccine—had also been shown to be safe. The risks related to the epidemic were potentially much greater than the risks related to the vaccine.

Another question was whether it was appropriate to seek to vaccinate subgroups of populations or entire populations. The vaccine may be safe and immunogenic, but this does not necessarily mean that vaccination is effective in reducing the cases of influenza, hospital admissions, and mortality. Indeed, group comparisons had not firmly established the effectiveness in reducing deaths or health services congestion of routine vaccination in subgroups of the population such as healthy adults of any age, health-care workers in long-term care facilities for the elderly, and children.[13] There was no evidence regarding the impact of vaccinating the whole population, but such major intervention can be expected to stop an epidemic by rapidly reducing the number of susceptible persons the virus can newly infect. When a sufficient fraction of the community is immune, the epidemic dies out.

Therefore, group comparisons contributed to the decision to vaccinate everybody.

Many objections were raised against the decision to mass-vaccinate. Some were mere beliefs. For example, it was argued that the vaccine composition, in particular the "adjuvant," was potentially harmful. It was claimed that the vaccine could cause a rare reversible paralysis called "Guillain-Barré syndrome" as well as multiple sclerosis and autism.

But these claims were of a different nature from the claims about the vaccine's safety and immunogenicity. This becomes clear if one asks, Were there group comparisons performed in human populations showing that vaccinated people were more likely to develop Guillain-Barré syndrome, multiple sclerosis, or autism than nonvaccinated people? The negative answer allows us to classify this claim as belief, theory, and opinion, sometimes built around laboratory findings, but not amounting to evidence of risk for human health.[14] No study in other primates, however close they are to human beings, and even if they involved an animal group comparison, can be considered as direct evidence of risk in humans. No public-health authority can base its policies on these beliefs or indirect evidence.

Fortunately, the H1N1 epidemic did not have dire consequences. Nevertheless, the Centers for Disease Control and Prevention estimate that in the United States about 61 million people got sick, 274,000 were hospitalized, and 12,470 died between April 2009 and April 2010.[15] But had the epidemic been more severe, these popular beliefs about vaccination would have dangerously obstructed the public-health strategy, increasing hospitalizations and deaths and overwhelming the medical response to the health crisis. This is also true for future pandemics, whose impact might be mitigated by mass vaccination.

One of the lessons drawn by the Parliamentary Assembly of the Council of Europe, which discussed the management of the H1N1 epidemic, was that "complete information needs to be provided to the public in a manner which allows even those with little scientific knowledge to follow the arguments in a dispassionate manner."[16] For this call to be more than wishful thinking, we "need" also to provide the public with the means to critically use this "complete information"—that is, to become familiarized with group comparisons, which provide an objective guidance with respect to this sort of decisions.

## TEACHING EPIDEMIOLOGY

The coming chapters provide historical evidence that the basic tenets of epidemiology (group comparisons and population thinking) cannot be acquired spontaneously. I don't see, therefore, how the citizen's right to be health informed can become a reality if the usage and interpretation of group comparisons is not taught in schools. For those who are already beyond their school days, continuous education can take care of this. Epidemiology classes are still unfortunately rarely given outside schools of public health, however. Throughout this book and especially in chapter 15, I argue that epidemiology can be taught to the whole population in a nontechnical way that overcomes some of the difficulties students encounter to move from individual to population thinking.

I have been teaching epidemiology to doctors, medical and public-health students, and health-care professionals for more than thirty years now. Like most other teachers of epidemiology, I have been struck by the psychological obstacle that arises when we start talking about populations, risks, and probabilities. Students' brains sometimes seem to freeze, and their gaze turns unexpressive. It is as if their cortex has all of a sudden been disconnected. There is nothing complicated about what we teach, but the mode of thinking is unusual.

I was therefore fascinated to observe that the psychological obstacle did not occur when, instead of teaching epidemiology using modern examples of studies, I began to tell how society came to embrace epidemiology to solve enigmas of health and disease. Since then, this is the way I teach epidemiology, for both beginners and advanced students.

I therefore invite you to tour the historical path taken by a science, epidemiology, and its migration in just a few centuries from the periphery of medical thinking to the center of the process of knowledge acquisition in medicine and public health. This tour revisits successive episodes in which epidemiology helped solve enigmas and unravel mysteries regarding main health and disease issues affecting human communities. This illustration of the considerable role that epidemiology already plays in our daily lives will hopefully spur the teaching of the interpretation of group comparisons to all citizens.

# 2

## PEOPLE, BUGS, AND EPIDEMICS

WHEN I ask a class full of students, "How long have human societies been plagued by recurrent infectious diseases that have periodically decimated populations?" the answer I usually get is "always." But what makes them believe that? And how can we know if human societies have always been plagued by epidemics or whether they experienced epidemics only for a limited and recent period of their existence?

I first need to clarify what I mean by epidemics of infectious diseases. Consider the flu or what we commonly call the flu—that is, a combination of rhinitis, fever, and weakness, which can be provoked by the influenza virus ("the" flu), but also by other viruses. We know the flu is an epidemic because it affects an unusually large fraction of the community all of a sudden. It then vanishes but recurs later. Classically, epidemic outbreaks of infectious diseases last weeks or months. But for some, such as tuberculosis or AIDS, the epidemic succession of surge, ebb, and fall can take decades or centuries.

### BEFORE EPIDEMICS

Large clusters of people can sustain the existence of microorganisms— bacteria or viruses—over long time periods by constantly providing new hosts to feed on. Consider smallpox. Smallpox-infected people, if they survive, acquire a long-term immunity against the virus and cease to be viable hosts. However, in an unvaccinated population huddle of approximately half a million, the smallpox virus is guaranteed to permanently find sufficient susceptible children. Therefore, if we can determine when in history the first concentration of more than half a million human beings occurred, we can assume that this may have been the first candidate population to suffer from epidemics of smallpox.

To discuss the evolution of human density on earth, let's make two simplifications. The first is that societies of biologically modern humans have existed for 40,000 years. The second is that a major change in the main mode of subsistence occurred around 10,000 BCE: before 10,000 BCE, human societies were essentially foraging; after 10,000 BCE and up to about 1800 CE, they relied mainly on agriculture and animal domestication.

Could prehistoric foragers, our human ancestors who lived before the agricultural revolution, experience epidemics of infectious diseases?

These societies subsisted for tens of thousands of years mainly on gathering plants and small animals, hunting, and fishing. They did not rely on either agriculture or husbandry as primary sources of food and clothing. The term *forager* has replaced the older denomination *hunter-gatherer*. It may stem from the French *fourrageur*, which once characterized soldiers who entered into enemy territory to steal forage or fodder. In foraging societies, gathering, hunting, and fishing are ways of plundering natural resources without replacing them. The wild environment serves as pantry. Foragers are nomads, moving to new places when the resources of one area have been depleted. The clans of nomadic foragers have therefore to be small—that is, less than fifty people in general. The case of the Bushmen !Kung of the Kalahari in the southern part of Africa has been popularized by the movie *The Gods Must Be Crazy*. Each !Kung clan comprises about twenty people who have rare contact—the moderator in the movie says once every two years—with other clans.

The early foragers were exposed to infectious agents.[1] Bacteria could infect wounds. Hunters could catch animal parasites when butchering wild game. Foragers living in tropical environments must have harbored parasites causing malaria, hookworm, bilharzias, and sleeping sickness. Periods of famine could have dampened immunity, leaving clan members susceptible to otherwise harmless microorganisms. However, foraging clans were too small and too mobile to suffer from recurrent epidemic diseases. If a case of a potentially contagious disease occurred, its transmission was limited to the members of the clan. If the clan was annihilated, the human parasite could not survive and thus could not become epidemic. If the healthy moved away, leaving the sick and deceased behind, they avoided contagion and ended the outbreak.

Another factor speaking against epidemics in foraging societies is that the great epidemic scourges that afflicted human societies from antiquity until modern times were caused by "new" human pathogens. Smallpox, measles, influenza, tuberculosis, and the plague are less than 10,000 years old and appeared for the first time in sedentary populations raising large animals. Dozens of foraging tribes have survived until recently in isolated regions of the world, such as deserts, African and Amazonian forests, and the Arctic. These contemporary foragers around the globe have provided sad evidence of their lack of acquaintance with the "new" infectious diseases that scourged agrarian societies.[2] They had no form of immunity against these epidemic pathogens. They were decimated by epidemics when they came in contact with infected modern humans.

Thus, in our current state of knowledge it is reasonable to assume that for 30,000 out of 40,000 years of existence—that is, for 75 percent of their existence—biologically modern humans were not threatened by recurrent epidemics.

Now, could our human ancestors who lived after the Agricultural Revolution experience epidemics of infectious diseases?

## FROM THE FIRST PLAGUES . . .

Things began to change around 10,000 BCE. Foraging was progressively abandoned as the main mode of subsistence. Human communities became sedentary, stored food, traded, and communicated with each other. They subsisted mainly on agriculture, animal husbandry or both. Populations grew rapidly. The threshold demographic concentration of half a million people was reached in Ancient Sumer (current Iraq) around 2000 BCE. We can trace the first of the new epidemics to that region.[3] Ancient texts mention pestilences suggestive of infectious disease epidemics in Babylon and Egypt around 2000 BCE. The epidemics of the biblical Exodus probably occurred between 1000 and 500 BCE. The plague of blisters (or boils) and the death of the first born—two of the ten "plagues" of Egypt—may have been epidemics of infectious disease.

In his captivating history of epidemics, William H. McNeill[4] explains that a second characteristic of agrarian societies, besides population density, set the stage for the emergence of these "new" epidemics: the close proximity between humans and large domesticated animals. Most of the bacteria and viruses responsible for devastating epidemics in human populations were animal parasites that adapted to the human organism. In the early times of animal domestication, animals were not isolated in barns. They lived among humans. In these new conditions, measles, tuberculosis, and smallpox migrated from cattle; flu from pigs and birds (we are still threatened by swine flu and bird flu); whooping cough from pigs and dogs; and so on.

Two counterexamples corroborate the thesis that both lots of people and domesticated animals were necessary to trigger epidemics. The first case is the absence of epidemics in Mesoamerica (Central America) before the Spanish Conquest in the sixteenth century.[5] Central Mexico had probably 25 million habitants by 1518, just before the Conquest, about 200,000 of whom resided in the capital of the Mexicas, Tenochtitlan, within today's Mexico City. Tenochtitlan was one of the largest cities in the world. Fatty dogs and turkeys were raised as a food resource, but there were no large domesticated animals such as pigs, cattle, or horses. The Codices, which described how the Mexicas lived then, do not mention epidemics.

The second counterexample is the apparent exemption of Africa from these epidemic waves. Its population density remained low because of subsistence modes based on relatively primitive and egalitarian forms of agriculture. The oriental and occidental slave trades resulted, directly or indirectly, in the destruction of approximately 40 to 60 million lives between the ninth and the nineteenth centuries. This human and demographic ordeal occurred during the period when epidemics increased in intensity and frequency in Asia, the Middle East, and Europe.

Thus, 2000 BCE is as far as we can trace back, historically and theoretically, epidemics of infectious diseases. Their geographical expansion after their probable appearance in Sumer is well described. Simplifying McNeill's ideas a little, we can distinguish four main waves.

First, from 2000 to 500 BCE, epidemics became routine in the large but distinct population centers of the Middle East, China, India, and the Mediterranean. Measles, smallpox, influenza, typhoid, dysentery, and dengue hit the same populations periodically but did not migrate across population centers.

Second, between 500 BCE and 1400, development of commercial exchanges facilitated the circulation of epidemics among population centers. For example, the Black Death of the fourteenth century started in Asia and spread rapidly through the Near East and into Europe.

In a third phase, between 1500 and 1700, transoceanic voyages and exchanges connected the populations of America with those of Asia, Europe, and Africa. While syphilis traveled from the New to the Old World, the then "childhood" diseases of the Old World—that is, measles, smallpox, mumps, diphtheria, and whooping cough—produced catastrophic epidemics upon reaching the New World. The population of Central America is said to have declined from 25 million in 1518 to 700,000 a century later due to war and epidemics of these new diseases.

The fourth phase goes from around 1700 to today. The oldest epidemic diseases declined in Europe. Plague disappeared and smallpox began to be controlled during the eighteenth century. In the nineteenth century, tuberculosis became the most lethal killer, but it was less disruptive than the recurrent epidemics of cholera that began to spread around the world.[6] After 1900, besides calamitous outbreaks, such as the Great Flu Epidemic of 1918, and emerging new human pathogens, such as the human immunodeficiency virus (HIV), epidemics of infectious diseases have not been chronic societal disruptors.

Thus, the idea that human societies have always been plagued by epidemics is wildly inexact. We have direct and indirect historical evidence of the devastating impact of epidemics of infectious diseases for no more than 4,000 years, or about 10 percent of modern human existence.

The emergence of epidemics of infectious diseases about 4,000 years ago provides a chronological milestone for the oldest possible age of epidemiology. There could not have been a science of epidemics before that. It is also about 4,000 years ago in ancient Egypt and then in Sumer that we can trace the origin of a medical profession.[7] If epidemiology had first emerged in Sumer after the first outbreaks, it would be as old as medicine, but it has taken thousands of years more for epidemiology to see the light.

## . . . TO THE TRIUMPH OF EPIDEMICS
## OVER MEDICINE

Thus, epidemics have been in existence for a period of 4,000 years more or less saddled across year 1 CE. But, then, during these 4,000 years how often were human communities devastated by outbreaks that killed massively and momentarily disrupted the functioning of society? Imagine a place in Asia or in Europe. Did major scourges hit it constantly every two years, every ten years, once in a century? Did the frequency of epidemics evolve across time?

To answer these questions accurately, we would need evidence about the burden of epidemics on people's everyday life since 2000 BCE. Apparently, no antique civilization monitored epidemic outbreaks within any region of the world for that long. We can, however, have a glimpse at the evolution of epidemics in the Chinese Empire, which lasted from 221 BCE to 1911 CE, because of two particularities of Chinese history. The first is that localities kept some sort of diaries of events at local, prefectural, and provincial levels. These gazetteers mentioned major epidemics among the events that punctuated life in these geographical areas, mentioning their place and time, but giving no real count of the number of casualties. The second distinctiveness is that emperors belonged to dynasties, such as the Yuan, the Ming, or the Qing. When a new dynasty came to power, the tradition was for the new emperor to commission the writing of the history of the previous dynasty. Gazetteers were used to complete this task, resulting in the recording of major epidemics in dynastic histories. In the eighteenth century, the Qing dynasty compiled the *Great Imperial Encyclopedia*, which comprised all of the dynastic histories.[8] Modern scholars have therefore been able to establish a catalog of "major" epidemics that occurred during the 2,000 years of the existence of the Chinese Empire based on the dynastic histories and the *Imperial Encyclopedia*.

My analysis of this catalog is summarized in figure 2.1, which shows that the frequency of epidemic was low before 100 CE. It stabilized at about

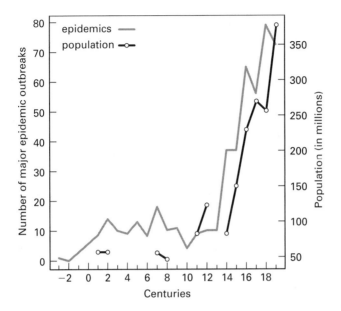

FIGURE 2.1  **Number of Epidemic Outbreaks
and Population Size in China, from 300 BCE to 1911**

*Source*: Morabia 2009a.

ten outbreaks per century between 100 and 1100 CE. Then, after 1100 CE it grew rapidly, reaching 80 outbreaks per century after 1800.

In figure 2.1, the parallel evolution of the number of people and major epidemics is fascinating. Like epidemics, the Chinese population, for which we also uniquely have demographic data over about a 2,000-year period,[9] grew rapidly after the eleventh century, even though there are two notable troughs during the Mongol conquests between the fourteenth and seventeenth centuries.[10]

Isn't it counterintuitive to observe that the more epidemics there were, the more people there were? Wouldn't you expect epidemic casualties to slow down population growth? McNeill explains, however, that the form of successful adaptation to infections, such as smallpox and measles, that the Chinese population seems to have achieved is compatible with both more people and more epidemics.[11] Toward the end of the tenth century, especially in the Yangtze Valley and regions farther south, these diseases infected most children but killed only a fraction. The children who survived had acquired a long-term immunity. Once adults, they could safely work, produce food, and have children, therefore increasing the population size one generation after the other. These millions of rice paddy farmers were able to colonize the vast spaces of central and southern China. Their productivity increased with early rice strains that could be harvested twice a year. They received an expanded share of the production. Because of better nutritional status and greater resistance to epidemics, the number of Chinese grew rapidly. But epidemics did, too, because each new generation brought an increasing lot of susceptible children to fuel their recurrences.

Thus, back to our questions about life with epidemics in the past, the Chinese example suggests that for most of their existence epidemics were far from being permanent concerns in everyday life. A further analysis of the evolution of epidemics in China, focusing on the periodicity and multiplicity of outbreaks, indicates that during the first century CE a family could live several decades free of outbreaks. Outbreaks became quasi-decennial in the sixth century. During the sixteenth century, there was an outbreak every couple of years. The same held true during the nineteenth century, but outbreaks were simultaneous and occurred in more locations.

The consistency between the demographic and epidemiologic evolutions in China makes sense. It is reasonable to think that the other large agrarian societies in Asia and Europe underwent the same adaptation. The development of an immunologic resistance to diseases such as measles, mumps, and smallpox also occurred in Europe between 1200 and 1500. When almost every adult in the population had acquired a durable immunity during childhood, children progressively became the only susceptible hosts, limiting the catastrophic, social, and economic impacts of epidemics.

The demographic collapse that followed the European conquest of the Americas is also paradoxically compatible with the Chinese experience. Estimates on the exact number of casualties vary, but scholars agree that the Americas (Central and South) lost more than 90 percent of their indigenous population, mainly to the "new" epidemics, during the first hundred years after Columbus's first voyage in 1492. Indigenous Americans, all of whom descended from a small stock of foraging men and women who had been able to migrate from Asia before the Agricultural Revolution, were highly susceptible to smallpox, measles, swine flu, and many other highly lethal plagues originating from animals unknown in pre-Columbian societies.

The triumph of the new epidemics in premodern societies of the Old and New Worlds is shattering. It is extremely shocking that after the twelfth century epidemics raged over the civilized world with increasing ferocity without meeting a force of concerted resistance. Against the rising menace of epidemics, all civilizations of the world were defenseless. Medicine was unable to slow down their progression. Actually, as we will see in the next chapters, in tracing the history of epidemics up to the seventeenth century, we can find virtually no historical evidence that doctors were able to understand their contagious nature, causes, and modes of prevention and thus to act against them. There is no trace of a science of epidemics. Why?

## GUNS, GERMS, AND STEEL, BUT HOLISM

Today, the qualifier *holistic* is commonly perceived as positive, whereas the qualifier *reductionist* is not. Especially when it comes to medicine. Holistic medicine examines the complaints of the "entire" person (*holos* in Greek means "entire"), whereas reductionist medicine focuses on the symptom or the diseased organ. Few people, however, realize that the modern qualifier *holistic* can also characterize medicine as it was practiced for 4,000 years before it became reductionist and that reductionism has been an indispensable step toward the implementation of group comparisons and therefore the emergence of epidemiology.

Let us therefore qualify as "holistic," for lack of a better term, the main forms of medicine practiced during antiquity and then from the Middle Ages until the middle of the nineteenth century in Europe, Middle East, Asia, and America. Even if the medical models and treatment techniques differed between the regional systems, they all considered health as resulting from an equilibrium, first within the individual and then between the individual and the global environment, which comprised everything in the universe. Health was lost when an imbalance occurred. But an innumerable number of factors could be responsible.

I concluded the previous section noting that the march of epidemics seems to have met no medical obstacle over 4,000 years. A logical question is therefore: Was it because ancient medical systems were holistic that they were unable to understand and control epidemics of infectious diseases?

During an epidemic, the proportion of people in the population who are affected by a given disease typically varies rapidly across time.[12] The emergence, peak, and resolution of epidemics can be observed only at the population level. Isolate a single sick person in the population, and the epidemic becomes incomprehensible.[13] And focusing on individual patients is precisely what the ancient holistic doctor did.[14]

Take the Greek doctor Hippocrates about 2,500 years ago. He was a wandering practitioner of a form of ancient holistic medicine. On his way to the village in whose market he would open his clinic, he would pay attention to the season, whether there were stagnant waters nearby, the exposure to the winds, and so on. He would inquire from people he met and maybe hosted him about how the rest of the year had been in terms of climate and health complaints. An apt astronomer, he could read the constellations formed by the heavenly bodies. Hippocrates was interested in environmental and meteorological observations insofar as they belonged to the many factors that allowed him to interpret each patient's symptoms and clinical history and predict whether the patient had chances of surviving or not.

Because all inhabitants of a locality shared the same environment, Hippocrates could have directly related these external factors to an individual patient's history. But he did not. Hippocrates did not think that epidemics were the doctor's business. When a deadly epidemic disease killed scores of people, regardless of their way of life or social background, the only resort was to flee the area or breathe more superficially. The doctors could not help. It was only when patients were afflicted by individual symptoms, reflected as an imbalance in their bodily fluids ("humors"), that a doctor was needed to reestablish the proper balance. Such doctors supposedly knew how to help the positive natural forces in the human body win the fight against morbid and lethal forces.

For example, examining a man suffering from abdominal pains on a cold day in spring, between the new moon and its first quarter, Hippocrates would have considered that these abdominal pains resulted from a combination of temperament, seasons, quarters of the moon, orientation of the winds, and several other factors that proved to be deleterious for that individual patient.

Imagine for a moment that you are Hippocrates and that during a full year of practice you have examined not only one but one hundred patients having abdominal pains similar to those of the man in our example. Had you counted, this is what you would have observed. If abdominal pains occurred just as often during each of the four seasons of the year, only twenty-five of the one hundred cases occurred in the spring. If the determinants of abdominal pain varied according to each of the four quarters of the moon, of the twenty-five cases of abdominal pains that occurred in the spring, about six cases (twenty-five divided by four) were influenced by the same moon quarter. Now, if one-third of the patients were bilious—that is, shrewd and prompt to anger—there were only two patients (six divided by three) out of the original one hundred who shared the same combination of factors associated with season, moon, and temperament. If, finally, it also mattered whether the wind blew from the north as opposed to another cardinal point, the last two patients would also belong to different categories. You could still consider diet, occupation, heredity, and so on, but already with four factors there is only one of the one hundred patients who was bilious and whose abdominal pains occurred in spring, between the new moon and its first quarter, and when the wind was blowing from the north. This patient deserved individual diagnosis, prognosis, and eventually treatment. This is precisely why Hippocrates did not count and saw no interest in it.

Thus, in his ambition to connect elements, celestial bodies, cardinal locations, organs, climates, seasons, colors, tastes, body fluids, and even expressions such as laughter or pain to explain someone's health complaint, the ancient holistic doctor had necessarily to focus on the individual patient. He could not learn and describe what happened at the population level. He could not consider that patients, even when they presented with similar symptoms, suffered from the same "disease." It made no sense to group patients into diagnostic categories, count them, and compute averages and proportions. The Hippocratic treatises always described patients one by one.[15]

Apparently, it is very different to treat dysentery using acupuncture and moxibustion as Chinese physicians did than to treat it using bloodletting,

laxatives, and purging as European doctors did. But the underlying rationale for these two sorts of treatment is the same: to reestablish the lost
equilibrium within the body. Purgation and phlebotomy were intended
to eliminate unhealthy humors; needles and moxa were used to balance
the yin and the yang.[16]

Both systems relied on similar rules of order and harmony governing
and structuring the universe, society, and the human body. Both systems
envisioned the human body as a small world, a "microcosm," which was a
mirror image of the big world, the "macrocosm." Compare two documents
written about 5,000 years apart in two different continents. The *Inner
Canon of Classical Chinese Medicine*, attributed to the mythical Yellow
Emperor of the twenty-seventh century BCE and compiled about 2,000
years ago, says: "A human body is the counterpart of a state. . . . The spirit
[the body's governing vitalities, *shen*] is like the monarch; the blood *xue*
is like the ministers; the *qi* is like the people. Thus we know that one who
keeps his own body in order can keep a state in order. Loving care for
one's people is what makes it possible for a state to be secure; nurturing
one's *qi* is what makes it possible to keep the body intact."[17] And William
Harvey's 1628 *De motu cordis* (Of the movement of the heart) states, "So
the heart is the beginning of life, the Sun of the Microcosm, even as the
Sun deserves to be call'd the heart of the world; for it is the heart by whose
virtue and pulsation the blood is moved, perfected, made apt to nourish,
and is preserved from corruption and coagulation; it is the household
divinity which, discharging its function, nourishes, cherishes, quickens the
whole body, and is indeed the foundation of life, the source of all action."[18]

The inability of all the ancient holistic medicines to move beyond the
individual and study what can only be observed at the population level
must have contributed to their failure against epidemics. Health knowledge about prevention and epidemic control stagnated for thousands of
years, even though during the same period these premodern civilizations
experienced continuous progressions in natural-science knowledge and
techniques. They had better guns and discovered steel. They got adapted
to germs, but holism did not allow them to understand that hygiene, clean
water, and mass inoculation could help controlling epidemics a great deal.
It is for this reason that the discovery of the New World in 1492 was both
a feast and a catastrophe.[19] Columbus faced the Atlantic Ocean onboard

remarkably performing sailing ships, including two highly maneuverable Caravels, but his spunky sailors unintentionally carried—among other epidemic-causing diseases—smallpox, measles, and plague, three diseases that cyclically killed tens of thousands of Europeans and would go on to devastate the New World.

## STRESS, DUODENAL ULCER, AND GENERAL GEORGE WASHINGTON

If agrarian societies understood how epidemics spread, would they have had the technological resources to attenuate the burden these epidemics presented? Most likely yes, because controlling epidemics in traditional societies was not a technological challenge. Keeping the rats away from humans would have helped to control the plague. Separating drinking water from feces and filtrating it in sand would have prevented typhoid fever, cholera, dysentery, and other causes of diarrhea.

Prevention of these ordeals would have required public cleanliness as the Aztecs had successfully implemented. When Hernán Cortes landed on the Mexican coast in 1519, Tenochtitlan, the capital of the Aztecs and their allied tribes, was an enormous, opulent city with canals, botanical gardens, and mostly artificial islands in the middle of a great mountain lake. Tenochtitlan was not only dazzling, but also (and probably most inconceivable for Europeans at the time) clean. An army of cleaners kept the crowded streets immaculate.[20] Unfortunately, cleanliness was not sufficient. The Mexicas did not realize that dumping the filth in the lakes whose waters they used for domestic purposes was responsible for the prevalent gastrointestinal disorders they experienced.[21]

Agrarian societies could have protected their populations from smallpox as well. Variolation—that is, the inoculation of smallpox material to prevent a full-blown form of the disease—had been a folk medicine practiced in much of Asia, Arabia, North Africa, Persia, India, and Turkey long before it was introduced in western Europe.[22] The Chinese, who claimed that the practice came from India, inoculated against smallpox via the nostril. When in 1718 Lady Mary Wortley Montagu, the wife of the British ambassador to Turkey, familiarized English doctors with variolation, it was already practiced in the Ottoman Empire. The principle of variolation, which seeks to strengthen the body's natural defenses, was conceptually consistent with the canons of holistic medicine.

Thus, the obstacle for controlling epidemics was not a technical one; it was conceptual and would last as long as holism dominated medicine.[23]

In 1637, the French philosopher René Descartes became a spokesman for the departure from ancient holism to a new philosophy, reductionism, whose key principle was "simplify!"

Foremost, Descartes advised that "to reach knowledge" in the natural sciences and in medicine we had to rely on observations and not on beliefs.[24] This "simplify!" principle was incompatible with all the odds and ends of ancient holistic medicine. The traditional speculations about the great equilibrium between the body and the cosmos or other astrological causes did not meet this new criterion.

The second Cartesian principle was that complex systems had to be broken down into simple components, which naturally lent themselves to observation and analysis.[25] The challenge was therefore to isolate a single factor among the many causes that the holistic doctor would consider simultaneously. This was the reductionist approach.

Francis Bacon, earlier, had promoted a new scientific approach strictly based on observation. But it was Descartes who stated succinct principles to support a new mode of knowledge acquisition.

Let us go back to Hippocrates's patients who, in the previous section, suffered from abdominal pain. This example illustrated why the "visual field" of ancient holistic medicine was inherently restricted to the individual patient. Consider now that you see the same patients, but as a modern doctor who adheres to the Cartesian principles of simplification and decomposition of complex models into their individual parts. Of the four possible causes of abdominal pain (patient's temperament, season, quarter of the moon, and orientation of the winds), you decide to examine one at a time. You isolate temperament and ignore, for now, season, moon, and wind. Wow! Your results reveal something completely different. Over the year, many patients with different temperaments develop abdominal pain. Some are bilious, and others are not. They come and see you under different conditions, but you do not bother to determine whether their symptoms appeared in winter, spring, summer, or fall, how high the moon was, or what was blowing in the wind. Temperament becomes the sole potential determinant of abdominal pain in a population of patients. You look at your charts and reckon that abdominal pain occurred among seven out of one hundred bilious people, or 7 percent. That's not many! This new information alone does not help. Abdominal pain occurs maybe at the same frequency in people who are not bilious. The reductionist approach has, however, transformed your visual field. You can do something that no holistic doctor could have done: compare groups. You return to your charts and calculate that 4 percent of the patients who do not have a bilious temperament complain of abdominal pain. You are now able to recognize that abdominal pain occurs more frequently among patients who are bilious. Thanks to your reductionist approach, you have a potential causal contrast for abdominal pain: bilious temperament, 7 percent; other temperaments, 4 percent.

The frequencies are not very high, and without counting and comparing it would be very hard to suspect the association, but the process of simplification and quantification finally provides a clue that a bilious temperament can cause abdominal pains.[26] This conclusion worded in old concepts becomes immediately modern by replacing the term *abdominal pain* with *duodenal ulcer* and the term *bilious temperament* with *stress*. The connection is biologically plausible: stress may increase gastric acidity and contribute to carving an ulcer in the mucosa of the duodenum.[27] Indeed, a study compared the risk of duodenal ulcer among 4,511 Americans followed from 1971 to 1984 according to whether they answered positively ("stressed") or negatively ("nonstressed") to the question "Have you been under or felt you were under any strain, stress, or pressure, during the last month?" The thirteen-year risk of duodenal ulcer is 7 percent among stressed people and 4 percent among nonstressed people.[28] These results are shown in figure 2.2

This causal contrast was not within your reach when you were a holistic Hippocratic doctor. Stress as a cause of duodenal ulcer cannot be assessed at the individual level. Take one stressed and one nonstressed person. Both can, by chance, not suffer from ulcer, masking the fact that duodenal ulcer is more frequent among stressed people than among those who are not. And even after years of practice, it is unlikely that a difference of 3 percent in risk becomes clinically perceptible.

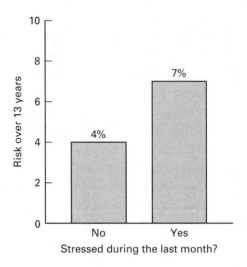

FIGURE 2.2 **Thirteen-Year Risk of Duodenal Ulcer**

Risk of duodenal ulcer among 4,511 Americans followed from 1971 to 1984, according to whether they answered positively ("stressed") or negatively ("nonstressed") to the question "Have you been under or felt you were under any strain, stress, or pressure, during the last month?"

*Source*: Anda et al. 1992.

Thus, the reductionist isolation of a single factor, temperament, led you to group patients into two categories, stressed or not stressed, which demonstrated that more of the stressed patients suffered from the same "disease," duodenal ulcer. Furthermore, it allowed you to compare them with people who were not stressed. Reductionism has stretched your visual field.

You are now ready for population thinking, like these pioneers of epidemiology, supported by enlightened minds such as Benjamin Franklin, who counted the number of deaths occurring among people who contracted smallpox either naturally or artificially though medical inoculation. They found out that natural smallpox killed ten times more than artificially inoculated smallpox.[29]

With the epidemiologic approach, you are now able to make bold decisions to fight smallpox effectively, as when General George Washington ordered the mass inoculation of the Continental Army. Most English soldiers were immune to smallpox. American colonists, in contrast, were susceptible to it, and their regiments disintegrated when smallpox broke out. In 1777, surmounting defiance from rebelling colonies and army hierarchy, the Congress authorized Washington to immediately and systematically inoculate its soldiers. "Thereafter," writes Arthur Boylston, "the threat to the revolution from smallpox was over. Inoculation became as much a part of soldiering as a musket."[30] The revolution might have otherwise been lost. The triumph of epidemics was finally trammeled.

## JIGSAW PUZZLES AND
## BARON VON MUNCHAUSEN

Descartes enunciated a third principle: ignore interaction between causes. When multiple causes are necessary for the occurrence of disease, Descartes suggested assuming that they can be assembled like the pieces of a jigsaw puzzle.[31] (See appendix 1 for a more formal description of interaction of causes.)

In holistic medicine, all causes interact because they are connected. According to my temperament and maybe the season, I will react varyingly to disease. The state of my liver will maybe impact my psychological state, which will maybe modify my sleep, maybe reduce my immunologic defenses, and maybe make me more susceptible to the threatening virus. . . . Each "maybe" is another interaction: it leads to a new health profile, which, ultimately, is unique to me and requires an individual therapy.

This is holistic common sense: body parts are not assembled like the pieces of a puzzle. Sickness affects the individual as a whole, not just an isolated organ. I cannot state that I am healthy, but my liver is sick. But the mode of reasoning that involves all the maybes splits populations of patients according to their individual histories and defeats any attempts to determine whether diagnoses are accurate and individual treatments are effective.

Confronted by a similar situation, the Cartesian doctor and many of today's modern doctors would say: let us treat the liver, then the psyche, then the sleep, and so on, as if they were independent problems. Let us rebuild the patient's health piece by piece. This strategy is frustrating for our common sense, but we know how to assess the efficacy of each of its component interventions.

Radical as it was, the third Cartesian principle targeted the heart of holistic medicine: the interaction between the doctor and the patient. The effect of a treatment cannot be dissociated from the context in which it is prescribed. Consider duodenal ulcer. The mere management of ulcer by an empathic doctor attenuates the patient's symptoms. In population studies of duodenal ulcer comparing an active treatment to an inactive pill called a "placebo," typically one-third of the patients receiving the inactive pill tend to improve anyway. This is the placebo effect. Unbeknownst to them, doctors must have relied on it for at least 4,000 years, back to a time when almost no effective treatments were available. The placebo effect has been to holistic medicine what shoestrings were to the mythical Baron von Munchausen. Doctors have been able to lift themselves out of systematic failure by pulling on the placebo string. By 1650, that was not sufficient anymore. The history of epidemiology was about to begin.

# 3

## PLAGUE'S SHARK TEETH AND SEAMEN'S ENIGMATIC EXHAUSTION

DURING THE first half of the seventeenth century, in the midst of a terrible period of war, famine, plague, and revolutions, Europe became the cradle of fresh scientific and philosophical ideas from people such as the philosophers Francis Bacon and René Descartes as well as the iatrochemist Jan Baptist van Helmont. These enlightened spirits were ready to dump ancient holistic complexity in history's wastebasket and start from scratch, using drastically simplified models. In their attempts to study the world objectively, they were overwhelmed by a mode of thinking that integrated everything, from the smallest to the largest, from invisible particles to planets. A worldview yielding a separate explanation for each possible health event was daunting.

Francis Bacon imagined a health research agenda designed to prolong human life by understanding the roles of heredity, height and weight, date of birth, food, diet, behavior, exercise, housing, and medical treatments.[1] Only common and manifest observations (if there were any)—that is, evidence—were admissible.

We saw in the previous chapter that Descartes's simplified vision of the world was indispensable to understanding what causes diseases and how to prevent or treat them. Four thousand years of medical history have proved that nothing—or almost nothing—can be learned about prevention, treatment, and screening from examining the medical records of a single individual or a comparison of two. Knowledge can be acquired only from another dimension in which populations are studied and groups of people are compared.

According to van Helmont's influential ideas, diseases were caused by environmental factors upsetting the functioning of the human body.[2] His vision shattered the foundations of holistic medicine according to which there were no diseases, only sick individuals.

The success of reductionism feels like a paradox. Today we value holistic approaches because they seem to fit better with the complexity of health and disease. And they do. Every individual is different, and holistic medicine is rooted in its fabulous ambition to solve each individual's riddle separately. However, it is a reductionist movement away from holism that gave us access to most of our current knowledge about prevention, screening, and treatment. Reductionism is justly vilified because it is a confession of ignorance: in artificially separating the body from the mind and in isolating the human organism from its global context, reductionism simply ignores what cannot be explained. This acknowledgment of ignorance is not sustainable. But in the seventeenth century it incorporated the key to unravel enigmas in health and disease: simplification.

It was in England during the second half of the seventeenth century that the new scientific approach was put into practice by the encyclopedic scholar William Petty and a population data freak, John Graunt. In *Political Arithmetic*, William Petty argued for a centralized statist count of men and products, a "statistic"—from a contraction of the word *state* and the suffix -*istic*—a form of systematic statewide data collection for bookkeeping purpose.[3]

## PLAGUE'S SHARK TEETH

Graunt was a surprising character, a fellow of the Royal Society even though by profession he was a successful businessman. Brilliantly taking advantage of the Bills of Mortality, which were early birth and death certificates uniquely available for London, he applied the ideas of Bacon and Petty to health. His book *Natural and Political Observations Made Upon the Bills of Mortality*,[4] published in 1662—that is, 350 years ago—is the first known application of population thinking in the health sciences. His work changed the perception of epidemic diseases.[5]

Epidemics in the seventeenth century had grown into a huge burden for social and economic life. Of all the deadly epidemics that cyclically hit London, the plague was the most disruptive. After the Black Death of 1348–1350, outbreaks of plague had recurred in Europe more frequently between the fourteenth and seventeenth centuries. These outbreaks put both political and economic life at risk. Wealthy people, politicians, magistrates, soldiers, and doctors left cities when the plague was present. The administration and the political institutions were paralyzed. There were riots and thefts.

The kings of England attempted to reduce the chaos provoked by each outbreak of plague by installing a surveillance system for plague deaths aggregated by parishes of the Church of England. Its results were published and made available to the tiny literate public. These London Bills of Mortality are the first known health-related population data. Old matrons, sometimes assisted by surgeons, identified the cases by investigating the houses where deaths had occurred. The local parish clerk routed the information to the clerk of London, where it was printed and sold on a weekly and annual basis. This activity became permanent after 1603. Thus, when those who were financially equipped to move away from London to the countryside learned from the weekly publication that plague deaths had been observed in the poorer parishes, they could organize an ordered retreat and, they hoped, contain the magnitude of the mayhem.

By the same token, the Bills of Mortality became available for analysis as a homogeneous series of health data. Graunt did something that no one had done before him. He designed a large data table out of the bills, with each row representing a cause of death, such as plague, smallpox, and so on, and each column representing a different year between 1604 and 1661. The table provided him with a perspective on the behavior of the plague in the population of London—a perspective no single doctor could have had. I have depicted the data from some of these tables in figure 3.1. Graunt was fascinated by what he discovered.

Graunt could not be surprised by the evolution of the plague deaths. Between 1604 and 1661, as per any Londoner's experience, there had been altogether twenty-seven years with fifty or more deaths from plague interspersed with years with only a few cases of such deaths.[6] There were years with plague and others without plague. Some outbreaks were horrendous.

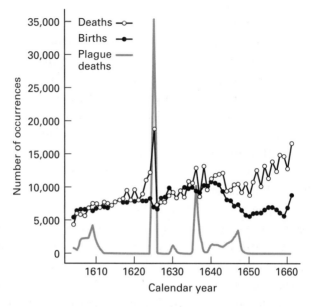

FIGURE 3.1  **Number of Deaths and Births in London, 1604–1661**

Evolution of plague deaths (*solid line*), of deaths from causes other than plague (*dashed line with circles*), and births (*circles*) in London between 1604 and 1661.

*Source*: Graunt [1662] 2004; Morabia 2013a.

In 1625 alone, Graunt computed that after correction for misclassified plague deaths, the plague had killed 46,000 people—that is, about 38,000 more than all other causes of death together.

The striking phenomenon, which the data tabulation literally revealed to Graunt, was the unexpected regularity with which most causes of deaths other than plague evolved. The number of deaths by other causes did not fluctuate from one year to another but instead maintained some consistency. This same regularity could be seen with births. In our modern minds, we take the regularity of mortality rates for granted. Epidemics are precisely deviation from that regularity. But try to imagine the perception of a seventeenth-century people who had never had the chance to look at tabulated data. They had the impression, as we do today if we rely on our personal experience, that births and deaths occur in an unpredictable way. If births and deaths are unpredictable at the individual level, why would they be predictable at the population level? Can you tell? Nonetheless, they were. Graunt observed that the number of births or the number of deaths from causes other than plague for a given year could be accurately predicted by their numbers from the previous years. There was therefore a sharp contrast between the irregular occurrence of the plague and the predictability of births and of many other causes of death. This observation suggested to Graunt that the plague had a different origin than the diseases that killed Londoners from year to year at a regular and predictable rate: plague had to be caused by some environmental factor that did not permanently exist in the community and that did not emanate, as for the "chronic" causes of deaths, from the "effluvia from the bodies of men."[7]

His conclusion debunked the multiplicity of beliefs, fads, and hype about the causes of the plague that circulated in his time. The dominant ideas were that the Black Death had been provoked by a certain alignment of planets and that it was transmitted by miasms, or fetid gases that emanated from the bodies of the sick and would seize susceptible people who inhaled them—hence, doctors' habit of filling long leather beaks with dry flowers and odoriferous plants and placing them under their noses when they attended plague patients. Yet none of these astrological, meteorological, religious, or superstitious causes could explain, as accurately seen in Graunt's statistics, why plague behaved differently than other causes of death.

Graunt's 1662 book sold very well and underwent several reprintings and editions during the seventeenth century. Did it have an impact on the disappearance of the plague, which occurred shortly after? The last great London outbreak took place in 1665. Was it a coincidence? Or was it that the quantitative description of plague epidemics by Graunt wore off the beliefs in astrological and meteorological causes and therefore led public authorities to impose quarantine more rigorously to boats and people coming from plague-ridden areas? Some historians have defended this hypothesis, but other theories involve change in the rat populations—we know today that rat fleas transmit the plague—and the replacement of wooden houses by brick ones, which separated humans from animals and rats more effectively.[8]

After 4,000 years of triumphant epidemics, the population perspective used by Graunt demystified the origin of the plague and generated knowledge useful to control this three-hundred-year-old, recurring scourge.

## WHY TWELVE BRAVE MEN TAMED SCURVY WHILE THOUSANDS OF OTHERS FAILED?

The term *population thinking* may give the impression that large numbers of people are required. But the population size is not the issue. We need just enough people to move from an individual to a population perspective. The Scottish Royal Navy physician James Lind (figure 3.2) proved it in 1747 when he demonstrated that lemons and oranges could treat scurvy.

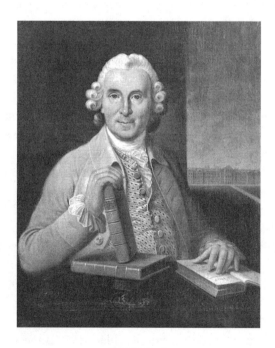

FIGURE 3.2

James Lind. Portrait by Sir George Chalmers. (From the James Lind Library)

In the eighteenth century, scurvy had become a major concern for the United Kingdom and its Admiralty. This scourge could kill more than half of a boat crew by a combination of deadly fatigue, friable bleeding gums, extensive bruises, skin hemorrhages, and swollen legs. It was an obstacle for waging long naval wars and conquering territories located weeks away from any shore. Scurvy destroyed more seamen than shipwrecks, foreign armies, and pirates.

The tragedy of Commodore George Anson traumatized the kingdom of Great Britain in 1744: most of the crew of five ships under his command perished from scurvy in an attempt to circumnavigate the globe. This maritime disaster stimulated research on the causes and treatment of scurvy.

Many people tried to find a solution to the enigmatic scurvy from their own personal experience, as the English mariner William Hutchinson did: "It has been my custom ever since to drink tea, twice a day, when I could get it. And to let lovers of tea know, I have made it in a very nice manner on board a ship. . . . With the above proposed method of living, I kept clear of the scurvy during the rest of the voyage, when many of my ship mates died with it . . . and have since enjoyed an uncommon share of health."[9]

Mr. Hutchinson was convinced he owed his life to tea. He may well have been right. Some teas contain vitamin C, and we know today that scurvy is caused by a diet lacking in vitamin C. But could Mr. Hutchinson prove that his two daily cups of tea were responsible for his good health?

If he were capable of traveling back in time, this would be easy. He would embark on the same boat, live through the exact same experiences again, but this time without drinking tea. If during this second life, he were to catch scurvy, all other things being equal, he could prove that tea protected him during his first life. Alas, living life twice is not an option.

Mr. Hutchinson had nothing more than an attractive anecdote about surviving scurvy with tea. Although he was convinced that tea protected him, his individual experience could not be generalized to other seamen. Mr. Hutchinson may have been protected by the vitamin C contained in the tea leaves, by something unrelated to tea, or simply by luck, but this we will never know. His opinion was a belief; it was not based on a find.

It is quite common to believe that changes in our behaviors are associated with subsequent changes in our health.

There is no solution to understanding Mr. Hutchinson's personal experience, but there is an answer to the broader question of whether tea prevents scurvy or not. Imagine a comparative experiment in which mariners free of scurvy, of the same generation and origin as Mr. Hutchinson, are divided into two groups. The members of one group drink two cups of tea per day while on a voyage, but those in the other group do not. Let us say that the two groups are so similar that it is not important to know which group gets the tea and which does not—in other words, the groups are exchangeable. If the seamen receiving tea suffer less from scurvy than those not receiving tea, we will be inclined to conclude that tea protects against scurvy. This find of the group comparison would have a strength beyond an anecdotic report.

These conditions were met on a navy ship in May 1747 when James Lind formed six pairs out of twelve scurvy-ridden seamen.[10] He gave all the seamen the same diet and stationed them together in one apartment in the ship's forehold but supplemented each pair with a different treatment. One pair was ordered to drink a quart of cider a day. Another was treated with twenty-five drops of elixir of vitriol (i.e., a diluted mixture of sulfuric acid, alcohol, sugar, and aromatics prescribed as a tonic for stomach disorders and sometimes for hemorrhages) three times a day. A third pair swallowed two spoonfuls of vinegar three times a day. (These acidic treatments were consistent with the medical belief at the time that scurvy occurred when marine air alkalinized the blood.[11]) Two other seamen were put under a course of seawater, about half a pint every day (no theory there, but what a potential boon for the Royal Navy!). The fifth pair received a paste made of garlic, mustard seed, dried radish roots, balsam of Peru, and gum myrrh recommended by a hospital surgeon. And the last pair ate two oranges and one lemon given to them every day for the six days that their availability allowed. There was no scientific rationale for prescribing citrus fruits, but it was common belief among seamen—and some scientists, too[12]—that they helped fight scurvy.

The oranges and lemons had a sudden and visible benefit for the two men who consumed them. After six days, they had completely recovered their health. Those who drank cider were better after two weeks.[13] The four other treatments were ineffective. Is it appropriate to qualify this small experiment as a group comparison? I think so because the logic remains the same whether the experiment is using 12 or 12,000 seamen. If one of the two seamen treated with citrus fruits had not been cured, the results would undoubtedly have been interpreted differently. It was a group comparison under experimental conditions as rigorous as the military ship permitted.

Lind was convinced he had discovered an effective treatment. He was not quite ready, however, to consider the lack of lemons and oranges as a cause of scurvy. He believed that scurvy was caused by both diet and, as professed by some great clinicians of the eighteenth century, the moisture of marine air. We know now that a deficit in ascorbic acid, also known as vitamin C, causes the metabolic disorder responsible for the signs and symptoms of scurvy. The human organism is not able to synthesize vitamin C, a substance that is very abundant in the natural environment but becomes very rare on ships once all fresh food has been consumed. Lind did not seem to make much of the fact that the pair who drank cider had improved after two weeks, but there was a clue to a protective feature common to citrus fruit and apples: citrus fruits are very rich in vitamin C, cider less so.

The Royal Admiralty was interested in Lind's findings, but when attempts were made to boil the lemons to get a condensed solution that would travel better aboard a ship than fresh fruits, the resulting lemon juice had lost its antiscorbutic properties. Heat destroys vitamin C. It took time to find the right formula. Fifty years after Lind's *Treatise of Scurvy*, the lords of the Admiralty introduced scurvy prevention by incorporating tons of lemon or lime juice into its seamen's diet—hence, the nickname of English sailors to this day: "limeys." At the sea battle of Trafalgar in 1805, scurvy severely handicapped the French crews but did not affect the limeys. This may have contributed to the victory of Nelson's fleet over Napoleon's.[14]

Thus, Lind succeeded in identifying a scurvy treatment with merely twelve seamen. Meanwhile, thousands of trial-and-error attempts of a variety of candidate treatments, performed by doctors on individual patients, without control groups, had failed for decades, if not centuries. The issue was not the population size in Lind's study, but the action of comparing groups. What Lind found was valid not only for the twelve seamen of the HMS *Salisbury*, but for most human beings, including Mr. Hutchinson. How many treatments from the eighteenth century are still deemed effective nowadays? There might have been many more had other doctors followed Lind's example.

# 4

---

# THE MYSTERY OF THE BLUE DEATH

## COLLECTIVE INDIVIDUALS

Imagine Adolphe Quetelet, a Belgian scholar of the nineteenth century, animated by a passion for population data, which he avidly collects. Quetelet gathers data from any source that he can. He obtains lists of heights and thorax circumferences of conscripts from military uniform contractors in Belgium, Scotland, Italy, and the United States. From registrar offices, he picks up statistics on marriage. And in some populations he even lays his hands on annual reports of crime and theft. He analyzes these data and is struck by the order hidden within these masses of apparently chaotic numbers.

For example, Quetelet plots each height value on a graph and ends up with a display of frequencies that takes on the shape of a bell (see figure 4.1).[1] He notices that the most common values are concentrated around the center of the distribution. And values that stray from the center mean values are increasingly rare. Amazing. Bell-shaped distributions had been known in astronomy, physics, and probability, but not ever for human traits. How is it that the bell-shaped curve could accurately describe a biological phenomenon such as height? Is there some order and meaning in thousands of observations made on a priori unrelated soldiers? What would you say? Quetelet's explanation was that there must be some divine intention to create a perfect man, the "average man," and all the individuals above and beyond the mean were accidental errors.

Also striking, the annual number of weddings and number of crimes fluctuated very little across time in his collected data. The number of

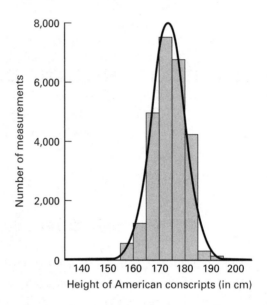

FIGURE 4.1 **Distribution of the Heights of American Conscripts Measured Around 1850**

*Source*: Quetelet 1869.

crimes committed one year could be used to predict their number for the following year. How come? Shouldn't the rate of individual decisions such as getting married and committing a crime be more erratic, less predictable? Quetelet saw society as the collective perpetrator, and the individual criminals or newlyweds as its arbitrarily selected agents.

Quetelet's are fascinating and difficult questions that still have no simple answers. Such data, however, did convince scientists that populations were more than just sums of individuals: they had genuine qualities beyond those of the particular individuals that composed them. We can visualize this idea in Eugène Delacroix's *July 28th: Freedom Guiding the People on the Barricades* (figure 4.2). This 1831 painting inspired some scenes of the Broadway show *Les Misérables*. It depicts a young woman with a naked breast holding a gun and a French flag and wearing the revolutionaries' Phrygian beret. She is successfully leading a

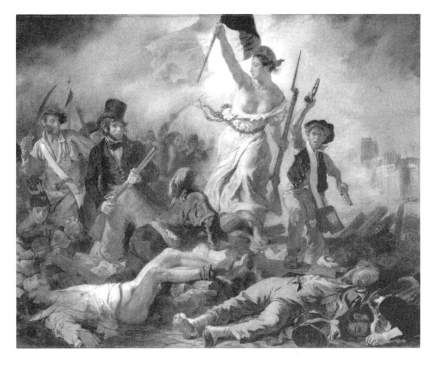

FIGURE 4.2

Eugène Delacroix, *Le 28 juillet. La liberté guidant le peuple sur les barricades* (July 28: Freedom guiding the people on the barricades). Paris, 1831. Currently at the museum of Louvre-Lens, France.                                    (From Wikimedia Commons)

miscellaneous troop of armed Gavrochian street boys, bourgeois students with top hats, workers, soldiers, peasants, and urban poor over the Parisian barricades that are littered with dead bodies (including the cadaver of a Swiss guard). We cannot understand the nature of this crowd by examining each individual in the painting separately. But collectively the street boys, bourgeois, workers, students, soldiers, peasants, and urban poor represent a sociological and political entity that has overthrown the old aristocratic and monarchic regime. This crowd has its own personality. Delacroix represented a collection of individuals becoming a collective individual.

This idea that populations behave like collective individuals is at the heart of many new sciences that emerged after the year 1800, such as demography, sociology, political economy, economics, evolutionary (Darwinian) biology, and statistics. These disciplines share the common characteristic of primarily studying populations as opposed to individuals. Populations can be regular and predictable, whereas individuals are not. This interest in population may have stemmed from the rapid spread of concentrated urban environments. Between 1800 and 1900, the number of US cities of more than 2,500 inhabitants increased twentyfold, from less than 50 to about 1,000. Moreover, the population of the budding metropolises grew: from half a million to 3.3 million in Paris, from 860,000 to 6.5 million in London, and from 60,000 to 1.9 million in Manhattan.

We can still feel the residual vibration of the explosion of ideas that resulted from the discovery of the distinction between the vagaries of individuals and the regularity of populations in the great theories and novels of the nineteenth century. The unit was the population. The scale was history. Consider the Darwinian theory of evolution and natural selection. Individuals who acquire a decisive reproductive advantage go on to form new populations or species, which replace older and endangered populations or species. Darwin's theory connects all living beings that ever existed on earth. Take the Marxist theory stating that the struggle between opposed social classes provokes profound changes of societal structures, from feudalism to capitalism and from capitalism to socialism. Classes are populations with collective individualities sharing common economic and political interests beyond their individual diversity. New classes appear, fight with the old ones, but are themselves bound to disappear. According to Karl Marx, his theory applies to the evolution of all human societies.

Epidemiology was one of these new population-based scientific disciplines. John Graunt's study of plague and James Lind's study of scurvy, described in the previous chapter, were seventeenth- and eighteenth-century precursors, but epidemiology soared after 1830. Its principle was simple: the cause of a disease or the efficacy of a treatment cannot be established from studying individuals but can be assessed from studying groups. The challenge was to find the proper strategies for studying a population.

## PUBLIC HEALTH

Public health is an intervention by the state aiming to protect the health of the public. It became a reality in the nineteenth century as well.

Since antiquity, states have invested in providing sewage removal, clean water, latrines, and so on. These public works were indispensable for the developments of cities, the historical nerve centers of civilizations. Large human concentrations required garbage removal, pipes, and roads, or else they became immense, foul cesspools. These state activities were not specifically meant to prevent recurrent epidemics. A telling example was reconstructed below the ashes in Pompeii: cesspools (*latrinae*), often situated in the kitchen, served to dispose of both human excreta and kitchen waste. In the absence of soap, food handled by contaminated hands easily transmitted dysentery or other gastrointestinal diseases, which were quite common. I mentioned earlier that the Aztecs kept their capital ultraclean at the expense of the purity of their lake water.

Take the measures against the plague adopted by urban magistrates of the Middle Ages.[2] They set burial regulations, banned the sick from entering the city, jailed any intruders, and sealed plague victims and their relatives in their homes until death. Only the rats and their fleas, plague's vectors, could escape. Magistrates ordained the killing of cats and dogs, viewed as potential carriers of the disease to neighboring houses. However, these animals also kept rats and their fleas away from humans. Repressive police measures were applied indistinctly to the plague and to criminals. They were not yet public-health initiatives.

Of course, some public interventions during antiquity can be viewed as "activity connected with community health," such as the availability of public doctors, but these actions were directed at individuals. They had a distinct nature compared with those proposed in the eighteenth century. Indeed, Johann Peter Frank, public hygienist of the eighteenth century, entitled his main work *A System of Complete Medical Police*.[3] Frank wanted health policy to regulate "marital hygiene," the manual labor of women, children's education, and hygiene in schools. Frank used, maybe for the first time, the expression "public-health legislation" (in Latin), stressing, however, that it was less important than alleviating people's extreme misery.[4]

In the eighteenth century, roots of a public health, qualitatively different from public "medicine," can be discerned, for example, in the isolation of the sick, the use of soap, and the inoculation of the Continental Army against smallpox. But things changed in the nineteenth century. Social reformers called for public works, such as sewage and garbage removal, in order to eliminate the sources of pollution that they believed caused sickness and death in the cities' poor neighborhoods. In England and the United States, these social reformers called themselves "sanitarians,"[5] from the Latin *sanitas*, which means "health." The qualifier *sanitary* was from then on associated with many activities of the state directly relevant to public health. There were sanitary laws and sanitary cordons, in which military troops prohibited population migration from areas ridden with contagious diseases. It was also in the nineteenth century that toilets were considered "sanitary" installations.

Sanitarians obtained the strengthening, expansion, and professionalization of the services in charge of collecting social and health statistics. Registries centralizing and archiving this information became data troves for epidemiologists. This surge of laws and actions and their beneficial consequences in the nineteenth century are the indisputable hallmarks of public health, an activity explicitly aimed at protecting the public's health.

## THE BLUE DEATH

After 1800, epidemics of cholera represented a new challenge for the nascent field of public health. This dreadful disease killed its victims, sometimes within hours, by radical dehydration from diarrhea, vomiting, and fever. When small blood vessels of the skin ruptured, they produced small hemorrhages, which gave the sick a black-and-blue complexion: it was called the "blue death."

The Industrial Revolution and the intensification of exchanges between the populated metropoles and their colonies facilitated the world dissemination of this disease, which until then had remained a local threat, particularly in India. A world epidemic, the cholera pandemic of 1817–1823, spread from Bengal, India, to Southeast Asia, Central Asia, the Middle East, and Europe, killing tens of thousands of people in its wake. Two pandemic waves occurred before 1850, reaching the Americas in transatlantic boats.

## THE CAUSE OF CHOLERA IS IN WATER, NOT IN THE AIR

In Europe and North America, it was widely believed that diseases were caused by particles emanating from rotten material that polluted the air and contaminated people who inhaled them. These particles were called "miasms," from the Greek *miasma*, which means "pollution." The major public-health figures believed in miasms. In England, William Farr, responsible for the collection and analysis of death certificates, and the social reformer Edwin Chadwick believed that miasms caused diseases. The German cellular pathologist Rudolf Virchow and American statistician Lemuel Shattuck also believed in the existence of miasms. Max von Pettenkofer, the great German hygienist, believed in miasms. These figures linked diseases with environmental filth and rotting matter and struggled to remove access to decomposable matter or to prevent its decay.[6] In 1885, for example, the New York City Bureau of Health declared that "Harlem flats have sufficient supply of rotting filth to generate fetid gases to poisoning of half the population."[7]

People who believed in disease-causing miasms could draw graphs showing linear relationships between filth and death. The filthier the place, the higher the mortality. The achievements of the sanitarian reforms carried out after 1830 in Europe and North America seemed to support their ideas. If cleaning slums, draining swamps, and building sewage systems reduced the blatant overmortality of the poor urban masses, was it not because these interventions eliminated sources of miasms?

In an 1849 report, William Farr even drew a beautiful graph showing that the higher one lived above sea level, the lower the mortality was from cholera (figure 4.3). The graph looked like a perfect pyramid with curvilinear sides, with a width that represented mortality rates from cholera and a height composed of varying degrees of elevation above sea level: the width of the pyramid shrank as elevation rose. Farr claimed that elevated locations had less cholera because the heavy miasms tended to stay low to the ground.

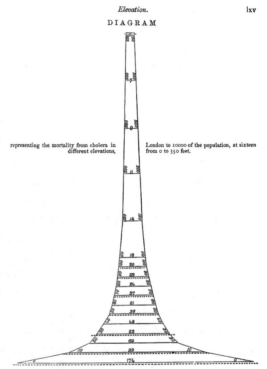

The figures in the centre express the number of deaths from cholera to 10000 inhabitants living
at the elevations expressed in feet on the sides of the diagram.
   The length of the *black horizontal lines* shows the *calculated* relative fatality of cholera in districts
at relative elevations indicated by the height from the base of the diagram.  The *dotted lines* indicate
the mean mortality *observed* in the elevations given. Thus:—in districts at 90 feet above the Thames,
the average mortality from cholera was 22 in 10000 inhabitants.

FIGURE 4.3

William Farr's 1849 graph showing the relation between mortality from cholera and
elevation above sea level. The magnitude of the mortality rates for the different elevation
levels are shown horizontally, occasioning the funnel shape of the graph. (From Wellcome
Library Images)

Miasms had intuition on their side. They fitted a simple equation: foul
smell, more disease; no foul smell, less disease. But the equation was wrong.
Fevers—a category that grouped many diseases, including cholera—were
in most cases not transmitted by air pollution. The sanitarian interventions worked because they reduced the propagation of still unidentified
contagious agents. This was precisely the theory defended by a handful

of doctors who posited that fevers were caused by some germ and were therefore infectious. When cholera, for example, broke out, preventing contagion required that sick people be isolated, ships and migrating populations be quarantined, and markets closed in order to interrupt the dissemination of the bug. But the theory of contagion was counterintuitive because one had to believe in the existence of small and still unidentified animals. Moreover, quarantines and other anticontagion means did not seem to stop the propagation of cholera. Politically, both the Right and the Left were opposed to them. For the social reformers, quarantine and case isolation were suspicious because their implementation did not fit into the reformers' struggle to improve the life conditions of the poor. For the merchants and shopkeepers, these means of prevention interfered with commerce and paralyzed business.

Had you lived in 1850, how would you have tested whether miasm or germs were the culprit of fevers? Both sides of the controversy used population thinking: lethal diseases were more frequent in the poor neighborhoods than in the richer ones.

If you chose to compare people exposed to miasms to others who were not exposed, you would find more cholera among those exposed to miasms and so incriminate miasm. Had you found that people exposed to water polluted with human excrement died more of gastrointestinal disorders and fevers than those who had access to clean water, as expected if the disease were contagious, sanitarians would have argued against you that it was because those drinking polluted water were also more exposed to miasms. There would be no way out except if you were able to conceive of a strategy to separate the effect of polluted water from that of air pollution. John Snow did.

## WHO WANTS TO BE A MILLIONAIRE?

And the million dollar question is . . . "Which English doctor of the nineteenth century is today considered the founder of two medical disciplines: epidemiology and anesthesiology? Joseph Lister, William Osler, John Snow, or Alexander Fleming?" You choose John Snow and win the game. John Snow (figure 4.4) has earned a spot in our general knowledge

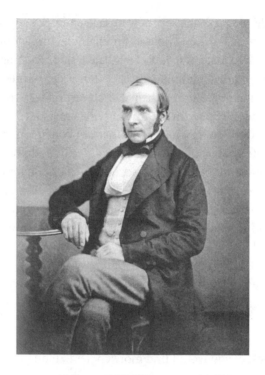

FIGURE 4.4

John Snow. (From Wellcome Library Images)

and deserves to be mentioned in games such as *Who Wants to Be a Millionaire?* As an anesthesiologist, he developed the clinical usages of ether and chloroform in his Soho practice in London. Queen Victoria asked him to anesthetize her during two of her deliveries.

During his medical training, Snow rapidly adopted the view that cholera was a contagious disease caused by germs colonizing human intestines. Healthy individuals ingested infected feces from contaminated hands, linen, or water, offering the germs new opportunities to proliferate. The feces released from these newly infected guts perpetuated the contagious cycle. Particular circumstances in 1854 related to the supply sources of drinking water provided Snow with an opportunity to test his theory using a group comparison.

In the mid–nineteenth century, Londoners drank water pumped from the Thames River, which flowed often unfiltered to their faucets through the pipes of private companies. The main water companies had their pumps in the center of London, but the Thames was massively polluted both by sewage dumped directly into the river and by the filth of London's harbor, which the tide cyclically pushed up to where the water pumps were. When cholera was in town, the water companies were, unbeknownst to them, the great purveyors of the disease.

In 1849, the British Parliament established that water suppliers had to move their pumps from the center of London, where the water was certainly soiled by sewage, to a place well outside the city, beyond the influence of the tides and therefore out of reach of the London sewage. The act was apparently unrelated to cholera. It appeased Londoners' complaints about the foul smell of their drinking water and its spurious solid residues. In 1852, one of the major water suppliers of London, the Lambeth Water Company, complied with the act of Parliament and changed the location from where it pumped water from the Thames. In contrast, another major water supplier, the Southwark & Vauxhall Company, continued to draw its water from a seriously polluted area.

Cholera was back in London in November 1853. There was a lull in it during the winter months, but then it returned in the summer months of 1854. For the public-health authorities, London was once again too dirty. In an attempt to quell the miasms, they purged the sewage and threw the privy contents into the Thames, along with the usual garbage, animal corpses, and other suspected sources of disease. And in doing so, they contaminated the Thames, London's river, and their source of drinking water. . . .

## A BRILLIANT IDEA

Snow had a brilliant idea. By moving its pump to a nonpolluted area of the Thames, the Lambeth Company had completed the prerequisites of a strategy to test whether cholera was a contagious disease potentially trans- mitted by water or not: when cholera returned in the summer of 1854, the Lambeth Company provided its clients with cleaner water than the

Southwark & Vauxhall Company. Furthermore, the scenario was such that some people had the same level of exposure to miasms. In some districts of southern London, the two companies fought for the same clients. It was not uncommon for the east side of one block of houses to be supplied by one company, while the west side of the same block was supplied by the other. Both companies' water pipes were laid side by side on the streets. On a map, it was impossible to clearly distinguish which company supplied which streets. In these districts it was therefore reasonable to assume that if a difference were seen in cholera deaths, it would be attributable to water and not to air pollution.

The only caveat was that Snow still needed to establish the water source for each household where deaths occurred. When cholera deaths began in July 1854, he immediately began his own fieldwork. From the Registrar General, he obtained the names and addresses of those who had died from cholera, went to their homes, and established which company provided their water. He gathered this information either by asking the people who still lived in the houses or by finding bills from the relevant water company. Snow also devised a chemical test to identify the provider on the basis of the tap water's mineral content.

During the first seven weeks of the epidemic, Snow attended his anesthetist practice in the morning and went to visit the homes of cholera victims in the afternoon. He counted 1,263 deaths in the homes supplied by the Southwark & Vauxhall versus 98 deaths among those supplied by the Lambeth Company.[8] Figure 4.5 shows that when he divided the number of deaths by the total number of households supplied by each company—information that was public—he calculated a ratio of 315 deaths per 10,000 household clients of the Southwark & Vauxhall Company and a ratio of 37 deaths per 10,000 households among the household clients of the Lambeth Company.

Snow claimed that the group comparison he had performed occurred under almost ideal conditions: no fewer than 300,000 people of both sexes, of varying age and occupation, and of every rank and station, from "gentlefolk" down to the very poor, were divided into two groups without their choice and, in most cases, without their knowledge: one group being supplied with water containing the sewage of London and, in it, whatever might have come from the cholera patients, and the other group being supplied with water quite free from such impurities.[9]

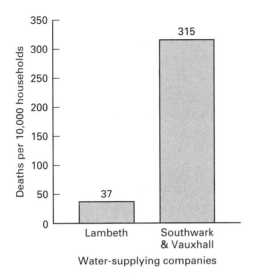

FIGURE 4.5 **Deaths from Cholera, London Households, 1854**

Lethal cases of cholera per 10,000 households living in London districts during the summer 1854 epidemic according to whether the water provider was the Lambeth Water Company, whose pumps were located in an unpolluted area outside of London, or the Southwark & Vauxhall Company, which pumped polluted water from the center of London.

*Source*: Snow 1855.

For Snow, exposure to miasms could not explain these findings because the urban environment of both water companies' clients was identical. Cholera appeared to be a contagious disease spread by contaminated water. Cholera transmission by air pollution had to be a false belief.

Snow also compared the mortality from cholera of the houses supplied by the same company in 1849 and 1854—that is, before and after the Lambeth Water Company had moved its pumps to cleaner areas. Mortality had remained constant where the Southwark & Vauxhall provided its polluted water but dropped fourfold when the Lambeth Water Company began delivering cleaner water.

Snow accurately described the enigmatic mode of transmission of cholera much before the cholera bacillus was identified as the biological agent of the disease. His population strategy unraveled cholera's mode of propagation and therefore ways to prevent new outbreaks. This knowledge has remained valid ever since.

Please do not get the impression that Snow's brilliant experiment resulted in a wide understanding of how cholera was spread. Most scientists kept believing in miasms until 1892, when an epidemic disaster in Hamburg led to the demise of this theory. Snow's opponents argued that he had not really proved that the houses of the Southwark & Vauxhall Company clients were equally exposed to the cholera miasms as those of the Lambeth Company clients and that, therefore, the two groups were comparable. Snow could only argue that air pollution had logically to be similar for people living in the same block of houses, but he had no data to rule out the criticism. Nevertheless, Snow needs to be credited for having devised the proper population strategy to distinguish between two conflicting hypotheses: Was cholera transmitted by air or water pollution? The strategy he used is the only one we know for testing conflicting hypotheses about causes of diseases.[10]

## THE PROOF FROM HAMBURG

Max von Pettenkofer (figure 4.6) is one of the greatest public-health personalities of all time. Brilliant and didactic, he was the leader of the Hygiene Institute of Munich, Germany, and, as such, had contributed to the transformation of his city, once disease ridden, into a healthy place. Pettenkofer was, for good reasons, an extremely respected public-health expert. Pettenkofer wrote numerous books, pamphlets, and articles on the public-health aspects of clothing, bedding, dwelling, air, food, ventilation, heating, lightning, building places, soils, and their relation to air and water. He had the clear style of a great communicator.[11] His downfall in 1892 was sudden and tragic. There are lessons to be learned from it.

### Groundwater-Level, High and Low

Pettenkofer straddled the controversy between miasms and contagion when he proposed a brilliant hypothesis borrowing from both theories and apparently reconciling them. He believed that the cholera germ released

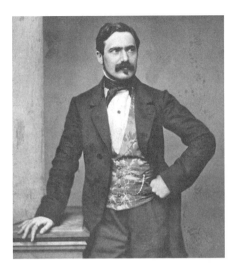

FIGURE 4.6

Max von Pettenkofer, c. 1860. Portrait by Franz Hanfstaengl. (From Wikimedia Commons)

from the gut of sick patients was harmless on its own. To cause disease, it needed first to be putrefied underground and liberated as a morbid gas, a miasm, into the atmosphere. Predisposed people who inhaled the gas fell sick. The quality of the soil played a crucial role. The miasmic metamorphosis was more likely to occur in the low and porous soils of locales immediately above sea level rather than in the rocky soils of mountain localities. Thus, Pettenkofer's theory combined miasms and germs in a single theory depicted in figure 4.7.

Pettenkofer's theory became popular in public-health circles because it seemed to explain contradictory facts that no other view could defend on its own. A transmissible cholera germ, but not a miasm, explained that the disease went from ship to harbor and markets before reaching more inland areas. But many observations did not support contagion until the cholera bacillus was observed using a microscope years later: Why didn't doctors, nurses, and other hospital personnel treating cholera patients always get it? Why were some localities more affected than others? Why did cholera outbreaks subside? Pettenkofer had a solution: look for the propitious soil.

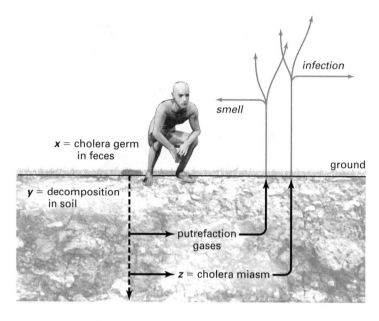

infection

smell

$x$ = cholera germ
in feces

ground

$y$ = decomposition
in soil

putrefaction
gases

$z$ = cholera miasm

FIGURE 4.7

Representation of Max von Pettenkofer's theory of morbid gas emitted underground: $x$ (the cholera germ) or $y$ (the quality of the soil) alone cannot produce the disease. If the distance from the ground to groundwater is short, $x$ will be transformed in smelly but innocuous putrefaction gases. However, if the level of the groundwater level is sufficiently deep, $x$ and $y$ will produce $z$, the cholera miasm responsible for the clinical syndrome called "cholera."

*Source*: Morabia 2007.

The germ is carried in human guts but cannot harm in the absence of a porous and dry soil.

The theory also had reasonable implications for health policy: in order to prevent the contact of cholera germ–bearing excrements with soil, there was a need to enclose sewage systems, isolate water for consumption and personal cleaning in pipes, drain swamps, and equip dwellings with floors. Indeed, cholera outbreaks occurred preferentially in poor and filthy neighborhoods wanting of such infrastructure.

Pettenkofer's theory was also seductive because it was analogous to the theory of fermentation of his French contemporary Louis Pasteur. Also a chemist, Pasteur had demonstrated that two necessary but nonsufficient conditions had to be met for fermentation—the process of synthesizing alcohol—to occur: a living organism and a propitious medium. Boiled (i.e., pasteurized) sugar cane juice did not ferment as long as living yeasts were not added. It was the same in Pettenkofer's theory: putrefaction gases emanating from soils (the propitious medium) did not produce cholera as long as they were not contaminated by the cholera germ (the living organism).

Finally, Pettenkofer's formula stating that $x$ (the cholera germ) or $y$ (the quality of the soil) alone cannot produce the disease, but $x$ and $y$ together produce $z$ (the cholera miasm), responsible for the clinical syndrome called "cholera," seemed to be directly adapted from the English philosopher John Stuart Mill's concept of "composite cause," according to which "the chemical combination of two substances produces, as is well known, a third substance with properties different from those of either of the two substances separately, or of both of them taken together."[12]

Pettenkofer's theory was only an untested theory—in other words, just a belief. It had not been tested using a group comparison. It would have been benign if it did not lead health authorities to make poor decisions. Pettenkofer was opposed to sand filtration of drinking water, to the quarantine of ship crews, to market closures, and to interventions aiming to prevent the spread of disease to other regions by migrating populations. He considered these interventions useless and expensive because they were not directed at preventing the cholera germ's contact with cholera-susceptible soils. But he applauded when people from contaminated zones escaped to the close-by hills and mountains and when businesses continued in the usual way. In reality, however, water filtration *is* an effective means of purifying it and thus freeing it of the cholera germ. Quarantine, case isolation, migration containment, and closing of markets can also prevent the amplification and dissemination of a local cholera outbreak.

How would you have assessed the validity of Pettenkofer's theory? Can you find some inspiration in the strategy Snow used to show that water was the mode of cholera contamination? For Pettenkofer, the quality of the soil was the key factor. His theory predicted that among two comparable cities located on different types of soil, the city located on porous soil would suffer more cholera casualties in times of cholera than the city located on rocky soil. Snow had already noticed that such a comparison would show that the characteristics of soils do not protect against cholera. Brixton, for example, suffered more from cholera than many London districts even though it was situated higher above sea level and with rockier soil than London. Can you imagine a design comparing two exchangeable populations in terms of soil quality and of exposure to the postulated cholera miasm, one being exposed to the cholera germ before it is transformed into a miasm—per Pettenkofer's theory—and the other not exposed to it? Hint: this is not an easy question.

## Hamburg Versus Altona

Here is history's answer. The population test of Pettenkofer's theory took place spontaneously in the summer and fall of 1892. This natural experiment had the most subtle design: two adjacent cities forming a unique conurbation with an administrative border in northern Germany, Hamburg and Altona, were located on the same soil, drew their drinking water from the Elbe River, and differed in only one aspect. Altona sand-filtered the water before supplying it, free of cholera germs, to consumers, whereas Hamburg, in agreement with Pettenkofer's credo, let the solid matter from the Elbe water decant in large reservoirs before carrying the water without further treatment to the city's faucets.

When the cholera epidemic of 1892 reached Hamburg-Altona and contaminated the Elbe River, 8,606 cholera deaths occurred in Hamburg and zero occurred in Altona. A mere street border neatly segregated the cholera deaths on Hamburg's side! Pettenkofer's theory was proved wrong. If miasms were the culprit, they would inevitably have crossed the border, and with them the epidemic would have spread from Hamburg to Altona. The mortality contrast could be explained only by the fact that Altona's habitants did not drink cholera germs with their water.

The rest of the story is unfortunate. Hamburg's health authorities, loyal to Pettenkofer, ignored the magnitude of the disaster and refused altogether to isolate cases, to quarantine migrants from eastern Europe seeking to embark on the Hamburg–New York sea line, and to close markets. A catastrophe ensued: 1.3 percent of the Hamburg inhabitants perished. Several weeks into the epidemic, the Prussian government forced Hamburg to trust the management of the epidemic to Pettenkofer's personal enemy: Robert Koch, a Berlin bacteriologist, who some years earlier had discovered the cholera bacillus. Koch came to Hamburg and imposed case isolation.[13] A few months later the implementation of a sand-filtering water plant freed Hamburg thereafter from recurring cholera and typhoid epidemics.

The groundwater-level theory had finally been tested by the comparison of the population of Hamburg, who drank nonfiltered water, with the population of the adjacent city Altona, who drank filtered water from the same river. The two cities were built on the same soil and breathed the same air. The only difference was cholera germ in one population's drinking water. The mortality had been 1.3 percent in Hamburg versus null in Altona.

## Koch's Achilles Tendon

Hamburg's disaster ruined Pettenkofer's theory and tarnished his reputation. In October 1892, in the aftermath of the disaster, Koch further humiliated Pettenkofer when he imposed his conception of prevention by disinfection and case isolation in the new epidemic law of the German Empire. Pettenkofer, who stubbornly continued to negate the possibility of direct contagion by the bacillus, fought back in earnest but was isolated and shamed. He was left with a single but risky opportunity to redeem his reputation.

The theory stating that the cholera germ alone sufficed to cause disease had a weak spot: Koch had never succeeded in causing cholera after inoculating the bacillus in healthy animals. All his attempts with guinea pigs, cattle, fowl, and rabbits failed. It was a problem for Koch because the successful inoculation of the disease in animals was one of the three criteria he himself considered necessary to prove the causal link between a microorganism and a disease. We can imagine Pettenkofer challenging Koch and saying: "Your incapacity in causing cholera in healthy animals comes from your stubborn refuse to take into consideration $y$, the soil factor."

"Or is it because cholera can only affect humans?" could have responded Koch.

"This is easy to check," did Pettenkofer say in substance. "Inoculate human beings with the germ, and you will know."

"Impossible, this would be too dangerous for the volunteers. Moreover, the clinical and public-health evidence is sufficiently convincing."

"Come on. Use me. I will be your human guinea pig. Provide me with a broth of virulent cholera, I will drink it, and you will see, I will not get sick," provoked Pettenkofer. "I will prove that the bacillus is ineffective if not transformed in the ground."

We don't know if such a conversation occurred, of course, but on October 9, 1892, at the age of seventy-four years, in order to prove that without telluric transformation, the bacillus alone was ineffective, Pettenkofer ingested a broth of cholera sent to him by Koch's assistant, Professor Georg Gaffky. To avoid the destruction of the bacillus in the stomach, he previously neutralized his gastric acidity using sodium bicarbonate. The broth caused diarrhea, and a microscope confirmed the proliferation of cholera bacilli in his gut. But, most important, Pettenkofer came out of the experience unharmed.

### The Missed Assassination of Pettenkofer

The ingestion of cholera was a heroic act that, for a moment, cast doubt on the validity of Koch's view but could not counterbalance the proof provided by the Hamburg epidemic. This last pursuit only delayed the complete victory of the contagion theory.

The reason for Pettenkofer's mild reaction to the ingestion of cholera remains elusive. Was Pettenkofer partially immunized by previous exposure to the bacillus? Did anger and nervousness provoke an extra charge of stomach acid that sufficed to kill the bacilli he swallowed? Did he develop an asymptomatic infection, which is much more common than symptomatic ones? Or did Gaffky send Pettenkofer a low-virulent culture of the germ, suspecting that the old man was going to ingest it?[14] I have discussed the latter thesis with modern cholera experts and historians: it is shaky. How could Gaffky have predicted the concentration and the virulence of the germs in the vial after they had traveled the 590 kilometers separating Berlin and Munich? Diluting a culture can actually stimulate the bacillary proliferation.

An alternative explanation would be that Koch sent the broth to eliminate Pettenkofer.[15] In 1892, Pettenkofer in Munich and Koch in Berlin were involved in a tough competition to control the empire's hygiene policy. The Berlin school won the two rounds: Hamburg and the Reich's epidemic law. When Pettenkofer requested the cholera broth, he added a third round to this academic feud. And he won! Pettenkofer's inconsequential ingestion of a cubic centimeter of pure cholera culture created a riveting fact that shook up everyone, including Robert Koch and Louis Pasteur.

Was the Berlin school prepared to lose this third round in order to save Pettenkofer's life? Koch did not have the reputation of being compassionate. Gaffky was closely tied to Koch.[16] For Berlin, Pettenkofer's death would fully discredit his ideas and definitely prevent new Hamburgs. Gaffky knew Pettenkofer would swallow the broth and therefore have up to one in two chances of being killed by it. To avoid Pettenkofer's death, Gaffky should not have sent the cholera culture, arguing that if the old professor wanted to kill himself, he should find other means.

We cannot rule out the theory that compassion guided Gaffky, but this hypothesis poorly fits the historical context and its protagonists. It can only be hoped that historians will eventually shed further light on this affair. Was Koch ready to kill Pettenkofer for the sake of science?

## The Causes of Cholera

Two years after Hamburg's tragedy, in 1894, the seventy-six-year-old Pettenkofer retired from active work. In 1895, cholera was successfully inoculated in animals. On February 10, 1901, a depressed Pettenkofer shot himself.

Where did Pettenkofer err? The problem was not the groundwater-level theory in itself. The theory was indeed wrong; however, Pettenkofer had correctly perceived that the cholera bacillus alone could not provoke epidemics. Cholera pandemics—there have been several since the discovery of the bacillus by Koch in 1883—have an environmental component, too. Here is how today's experts think it works. Intense episodes of warm precipitation in the Indian subcontinent transform the temperature and salinity of estuaries. The influx of large quantities of freshwater mobilizes stored nutrients in the bottom sediments and gives the dormant cholera bacterium a head start in its growth cycle. With the help of small crustaceans called "copepods," the bacillus reaches the gut tracts first of crabs, clams, and oysters and ultimately of humans who ingest the contaminated seafood raw and disseminate the disease to other humans. The epidemic then spreads rapidly until most of the population has been infected, with or without symptoms, and some die. The outbreak ends when susceptible hosts become too sparse. But cholera only fades away, hiding and cycling in estuaries until waning immunity against it allows a new outbreak. The Haiti epidemic of 2010 illustrates once again that cholera outbreaks result from the confluence of environmental, bacteriologic, and social factors, a sort of germ–environment interaction, which Pettenkofer had correctly perceived.

With hindsight, Pettenkofer's main mistake was not to test the validity of his groundwater-level theory with a group comparison before it put thousands of people at risk when tested in the Hamburg–Altona experiment. This was the true cause of his downfall. And here is the lesson: as attractive and apparently explanatory a theory may be, it is flimsy until it survives the challenge of a comparative population strategy.

# 5

## THE NUMERICAL METHOD

IN THE preceding chapters, we saw the powerful impact of group comparisons in separating knowledge from beliefs regarding the cause and prevention of cholera. John Snow actively showed that cholera killed more clients of the water company that pumped polluted water than clients of the company that pumped clean water. Max von Pettenkofer failed to rely on a comparative experiment, but during the epidemic of 1892 the citizens of Hamburg, whose water came unfiltered from the river, were badly affected by cholera, whereas the citizens of Altona, who drank filtered water, were totally spared.

Thus, comparing groups of people to establish health knowledge became the hallmark of an emerging public-health discipline: epidemiology. In this chapter, we will see that in the nineteenth and early twentieth centuries, epidemiology also came to the rescue of clinical medicine to evaluate the established modes of treatment and controlling nosocomial epidemics.

Before epidemiology, the medical profession had no tool to assess the efficacy of its treatments. Around 1830, consistent with the ancient holistic tradition, treatments were still tailored to each patient. Doctors would have found it absurd to group patients having received a similar drug or intervention to determine if one treatment was more successful than others.

### BARTLEY'S APOTHECARY COUNTS

The second cholera pandemic, which began in India, broke out in New York in 1832. The city already had about 250,000 inhabitants, concentrated mostly below Fourteenth Street. Of the 3,515 people who died during the epidemic, many came from Five Points, a crowded slum of African Americans and Irish immigrants north of City Hall. We can imagine Five Points as Martin Scorsese reconstituted it in *Gangs of New York*, except that in the movie the initial battle between the Irish and the "natives" took place about fifteen years later.

We owe to Horatio Bartley, an apothecary, a pamphlet of illustrations and descriptions of cholera cases at one of the New York City hospitals.[1] Bartley's document provides remarkable insight into the medical management of cholera patients. His observations were made in New York, but he would have observed the same thing in Paris, Vienna, or London. Of the 410 patients admitted to this hospital, 179 died. This is compatible with what we know today: cholera used to kill one out of every two patients then.

In his pamphlet, Bartley draws portraits of some patients,[2] indicates the treatment each received, and notes the treatment's outcome. For example, J.G., thirty-one years old, admitted in preshock condition, received mercury, sulfur, and anodyne enema, and died. P.S., thirty-three, Negro, also admitted in preshock condition, died. E.W., forty-three, Irish, admitted in preshock condition, received mercury hot toddy to drink, and died. H.W., fifty-six, from Barbados, received dry frictions, camphor, sweet oil, oil of peppermint, and ammonia and died. M.W., New Yorker, received camphor, "black drops," and mercury and survived! But when the latter treatment was given to E.W., he died.

How did doctors choose which treatment to give to which patients? The therapeutic cocktail differed for almost every patient. As a good apothecary, Bartley counted the hundreds of patients admitted during the 1832 cholera outbreak. However, it did not occur to him, or to anyone else, to group them and compare their mortality according to whether their treatment contained mercury, camphor, or peppermint. He would have noticed that half of the patients died whatever treatment they received and that therefore none of the treatments worked.

Without group comparison, there was a limit to what medicine could learn from the management of cholera patients during the 1832 epidemic. In contrast to the wasted opportunity of the 1832 cholera outbreak, valid medical knowledge was acquired when the treatments of pneumonia and puerperal fever were evaluated using group comparisons. Cholera, pneumonia, and puerperal fever belonged to the wider category of fevers.

## BLOODLETTING, A THERAPEUTIC PILLAR MADE OF CLAY

The emergence in the nineteenth century of large medical hospitals, with bed concentrations reaching the thousands, created the first opportunity for doctors to view patients as part of a greater whole, a population. Doctors were therefore able to assess the success of their clinical practice using a population strategy that became known as the "numerical method." The idea was that comparing groups of patients gave the solution to medical questions that could not be addressed by the clinical examination of individual patients, however numerous these individual observations might be.

During the 1830s and 1840s, almost all patients admitted for a fever to Parisian or Bostonian hospitals were likely to receive at least one, but very often all three of the therapeutics remnant of the still holistic medicine: bloodletting, emetics, and laxatives. We know today that these treatments were based on the false assumption that they reestablished a ruptured humoral equilibrium in the patient's organism. None of them really worked. It is therefore remarkable to see that they had dominated medical practice in Europe for more than 2,000 years and were deeply entrenched in doctors' practice.

After 1789, the French Revolution, which had vowed to make a clean sweep of the old-regime medicine, did not debase the three therapeutic pillars, but there were attempts to simplify them. For example, François Joseph Victor Broussais, a charismatic and influential Parisian doctor and a Jacobin who served in the Napoleonic army, proposed to make bloodletting the universal treatment for all inflammatory diseases.[3] Bleeding a patient consisted of cutting a vein and releasing several pints of blood or using leeches to suck the patient's blood from the region of the diseased organ. Leeches were preferred for localized inflammation, whereas venosection was used for generalized inflammation during which the patient would become ruddy and feverish with a fast and strong pulse.

The number of leeches procured for medical purposes totaled in the tens of millions in France and England[4] and in the hundreds of millions in Europe as a whole.[5]

For many doctors, Broussais's ideas brought order into a therapeutic mess by eliminating many treatments that utilized obscure mechanisms, were usually ineffective, and were too often toxic.[6] Some doctors, however, were not convinced that bleeding had any beneficial effect, and among them was Pierre Charles Alexandre Louis (figure 5.1). As a young doctor, he had traveled to the Ukraine and practiced medicine in Odessa, where he realized how insufficient medical knowledge was. In 1820, he returned to Paris, where during seven years of intense clinical activity at the Parisian hospital La Charité he systematically examined all patients admitted and eventually performed the necropsy of all who died. For each of them, he recorded on a card the clinical presentation, the treatment, and, when

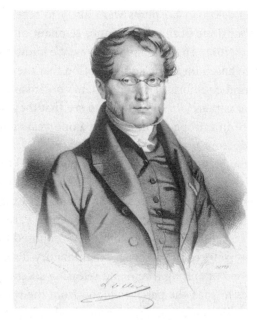

FIGURE 5.1

Pierre Charles Alexandre Louis. Lithograph by Maurin. (From Wikimedia Commons)

applicable, the necropsy findings. Louis accrued about 2,000 cards and used them to write groundbreaking clinical descriptions of tuberculosis[7] and typhoid fever.[8]

Louis's ideas led him to challenge Broussais's theory about the efficacy of bleeding in the treatment of various "inflammatory" diseases. One of these diseases was pneumonia, which was believed to be caused by an inflammation of the lung and was often referred to as "pneumonitis." Louis asked: "What is to be done in order to know whether bloodletting has any favorable influence on pneumonia and the extent of that influence?" Had you been in Louis's shoes, what would you have done? A logical solution would be to compare the survival of patients suffering from pneumonia who were bled with that of patients who had not been bled. The problem was that all seventy-seven patients in Louis's collection of clinical cards who had been admitted for a form of pneumonia that typically began with a huge, body-shaking shiver had been bled.[9] The only difference among the patients was that some had been bled immediately after the occurrence of the characteristic peak of fever and acute shivering (within the first four days of being ill), whereas others had been bled starting five to nine days after the onset of the disease.

Louis opted "to ascertain whether, other things being equal, the patients who were bled on the first, second, third or fourth day of their illness, recovered more readily than those bled at a later period."[10] He devised a strategy to test exactly that.

As shown in figure 5.2, more patients (44 percent) had died out of the forty-one who were bled early on than out of the thirty-six who were bled five days or more into the illness (25 percent).[11] Bleeding did not have the strong protective effect Broussais expected. It could even be seen in his results that bleeding might have aggravated the course of the disease.

Comparing groups of patients was at the core of Louis's numerical method and how he carried out his study. Louis started with seventy-seven pneumonic patients. The group comparison was naive, and this was reflected in the fact that there were several ways to perform it. He chose to compare those who were bled shortly after the onset of the disease with those who were bled days into the progression of their pneumonia. He could have also compared the fifty who had survived the disease with the twenty-seven patients who had not. Louis insisted on the fact that

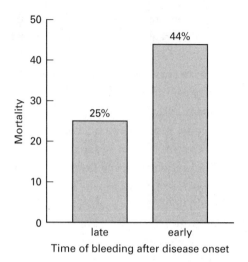

FIGURE 5.2 **Bloodletting and Deaths from Pneumonia, Paris 1828**

Proportion of deaths (percentage) of patients suffering from pneumonia according to whether they were bled between the first and the fourth day after the beginning of pneumonia ("early") or between the fifth and the ninth day after the beginning of pneumonia ("late").

*Source*: Louis 1836.

mortality was 44 percent among those bled early versus 25 percent among those bled late. He could also have stressed that among the dead 67 percent had been bled early, and among those who survived 46 percent had been bled early. It did not really matter which comparison he preferred. This naïveté made his argument less compelling and explains, at least in part, the little impact he had on French medicine during his lifetime.

Louis's work has become legendary, and, as in all legends, the tale told departs from the true story. A first legend says that Louis advocated abolishing the medical usage of bleeding. In reality, Louis simply showed that bleeding did not work as well as typically thought. He claimed that bloodletting was a therapeutic pillar made of clay. In the 1830s, such a statement was revolutionary.[12] It was only fifty years later that the bacterial origin of the type of pneumonia of Louis's cases was established. But Louis's fundamental historical contribution, which still sounds modern to us, is that even the most entrenched treatments may be proved ineffective if rigorously evaluated using a comparative population strategy.

Another legend is that Louis was the "first" to implement group comparisons in clinical practice. In truth, English doctors had already had the idea of analyzing hospital data toward the end of the eighteenth century.[13] Military and civilian hospitals, infirmaries, and outpatient facilities for ambulant patients were an outstanding feature of the British health-care system under the reign of George III. The registries of these institutions of mass medicine were for doctors what the Bills of Mortality had been for John Graunt: a source of clinical and pathological data ready for statistical analysis. The information accumulated in these databases was more voluminous than what any individual practitioner could accrue in a lifetime. Louis's contribution is more widely known today than that of his predecessors, however, because he debunked bleeding, which most doctors considered, along with emetics and enemas, indispensable in their therapeutic armamentarium.

The scandal raised by Louis's conclusions helped popularize the usage of group comparisons to assess the potential harms and benefits of a treatment. His approach opened considerable opportunities for acquiring medical knowledge. It made knowledge possible where the clinical approach, one patient at a time, was inefficient. The simple idea of grouping patients was provocative in 1830.[14] But the insistent Louis put his ideas into practice and brilliantly promoted them. His work was timely. It arrived at the right moment to justly contradict medical beliefs.

Louis had numerous disciples in Europe and the United States. Many of them influenced public health in the nineteenth century and proudly claimed to have been his student.[15] A century later, the discipline of clinical epidemiology and the concept of evidence-based medicine could trace their roots to Louis's legacy.

## HOW COULD DOCTORS RESIST WASHING THEIR HANDS BEFORE DELIVERIES FOR HALF A CENTURY?

The emergence of large populations of patients admitted into hospitals in the nineteenth century also opened up new opportunities to evaluate medical care, as illustrated by the process of eventually preventing puerperal fever, a historic although tragic milestone. This devastating disease affected healthy women within the first three days after labor and childbirth. It progressed rapidly, causing severe abdominal pain, fever, exhaustion, and death. The feverish mothers were often bled. Hospital outbreaks appeared at the end of the eighteenth century in France, England, and Austria and increased rapidly thereafter. Bizarrely, outbreaks were more frequent and severe in first-rate hospitals.

Indeed, outbreaks had hit almost unremittingly between 1820 and 1848 the General Hospital of Vienna, one of the largest and most modern hospitals in the world. Medical students came from everywhere to receive there the latest form of education combining bedside training and anatomopathology. For example, young obstetricians would examine and deliver women at the clinic and dissect the cadavers of those who died, in particular of puerperal fever. In the process, they learned to relate clinical observations with morphological changes in the body and the diseased organs.

The General Hospital also collected statistics about its patients. Ignaz Philipp Semmelweis, a Hungarian physician in charge of the obstetrical clinic, was extremely concerned by the differences in overall mortality between the hospital's two obstetric clinics. In Clinic 1, male obstetricians and medical students performed deliveries and eventually autopsied any mothers who died during labor. Clinic 2 was staffed by midwives only, who did not practice autopsies. Except for a small number of women requiring special medical attention, young pregnant women were directed to one of the two clinics according to their day of admission.[16] The hospital statistics showed that maternal mortality was two to four times higher in Clinic 1 than in Clinic 2. In 1846, mortality was approximately 11.4 percent—one out of every ten delivered women—in the General Hospital's medical clinic, versus 2.7 percent in the midwife clinic.[17]

Given the mode of allocation of the young mothers to the two clinics, social class or health status must have been similar among the women whose deliveries the doctors performed and those whose deliveries the midwives performed. Why was the mortality so different? Doctors believed that the disease affecting the new mothers was caused by a combination of individual predispositions and cosmic, atmospheric, and environmental influences. The hospital had tried, without effect, to improve ventilation and sunlight in the delivery rooms to reduce the miasms.

What could be the culprit? Today, 150 years later, despite what you may know about this episode, how would you have proceeded to try and identify a potential flaw in the medical care?

For Semmelweis, the eye-opening event was the death of a colleague anatomopathologist from a clinical syndrome resembling puerperal fever after he sustained a scalpel cut during an autopsy. Semmelweis grasped that there could be some connection between the disease and the pathological dissections of cadavers that were carried out by physicians immediately before moving on to examine young mothers and performing deliveries. But how? Some doctors may have washed their hands with water and maybe soap after having performed autopsies. The doctors at the time were no better or worse than those today. They were sensible enough not to carry macroscopic cadaveric material into the delivery rooms. Some of the parturient women were their own relatives and friends. For anyone who believed that puerperal fever was caused by miasms or other environmental factors, there was nothing wrong in the way medical care at the General Hospital was conducted.

Semmelweis had a second key intuition. Even when washed with soap, the doctors' hands exuded a cadaveric smell when the doctors officiated in the delivery room. Semmelweis speculated that the smell came from invisible "cadaveric particles" from the autopsy room that doctors carried on their hands, with which they contaminated the young women. After all, performing autopsies was the only difference between the clinic serviced by midwives and the one serviced by doctors. Semmelweis therefore searched for a washing solution that could eliminate the smell. He found that chlorinated lime worked. What he could not suspect is that bleaching the doctor's hand with chlorinated lime had sufficient antiseptic properties to kill the (still undiscovered) bacteria that caused puerperal fever. Driven by the right theory, he had succeeded in devising the right preventive approach.

At the end of May 1847, Semmelweis forced his interns to wash off the cadaveric smell from their hands using a solution of chlorinated lime before examining women. The interns reared up and disputed the orders, which they did not understand, but finally obeyed when faced by

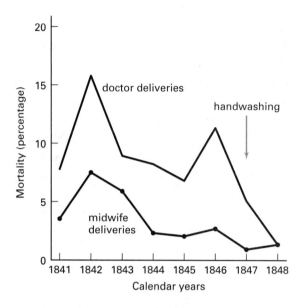

FIGURE 5.3 **Deaths of Mothers After Delivery, Vienna, 1841–1848**

Evolution of the proportion of mothers' deaths following deliveries at the doctor-operated Clinic 1 and at the midwife-operated Clinic 2 of the General Hospital of Vienna before and after Ignaz Semmelweis's introduction of compulsive hand bleaching with a solution of chlorine and lime in 1847.

*Source:* Carter 1983.

an intransigent Semmelweis. Figure 5.3 shows that during the following weeks, maternal mortality dropped to 1.3 percent of all deliveries, a proportion similar to that observed in the midwife clinic.

The obstetricians' tainted hands were the culprit behind the maternal overmortality in the doctor's clinic. During vaginal examination and delivery, doctors contaminated young and healthy mothers with infectious material that they unknowingly carried on their hands after the necropsy of infected women. In retrospect, it was shown that the outbreaks of puerperal fever began in 1823, when anatomopathology was introduced, and declined rapidly in 1847, when Semmelweis introduced chlorine into the washing routine.[18]

Semmelweis performed a group comparison. One group comprised pregnant women attended to by doctors, and the other group pregnant women attended to by midwives. The two groups were probably similar in many aspects because the selection into one group or the other depended merely on the day of admission, not on some independent characteristic of the mother. Semmelweis compared the change in mortality from puerperal fever before and after the introduction of chlorinated lime. Between 1847 and 1848, it declined from 5 percent to 1.3 percent of all deliveries, whereas for the women attended by midwives it remained constant at about 1 percent.

Semmelweis's conclusion was predicated on the similarity of the populations attending the two clinics. It is reasonable to think that the allocation to each clinic by day of admission made their populations quite similar. Nevertheless, the medical clinic received four to five hundred more patients per year, plus women requiring special medical care. To address this criticism, a finer study than Semmelweis's would have been needed, in which only the women requiring normal care would have been compared.

I admit that the heading for this section is provocative. Doctors did not "resist washing their hands." They refused the ridicule that came along with succumbing to the fad of believing in "cadaveric particles." As long as Semmelweis's ideas were only ideas, the doctors' skepticism about "disinfection" was warranted. They failed, however, to understand that by using a comparative intervention (washing off the smell), Semmelweis had effectively evaluated the obstetrical care and solved the enigma of puerperal fever decades before the "particles" were finally seen under a microscope.

Semmelweis's group comparison tested a simple causal question: Do hands stained with cadaveric particles transmit puerperal fever? It generated more knowledge about this disease than hundreds of thousands of clinical examinations of individual patients.

There is a fascinating side question to Semmelweis's story. Did the Viennese population suspect a link between puerperal fever and the medical Clinic 1 before doctors did? Apparently, it was not uncommon for women to delay the day and time of their hospital admission in order to be admitted to the midwife-operated Clinic 2. When the medical Clinic 1 was in charge, five or six women per day preferred to give birth in the street or in a field and to come to the hospital with their newborn in their hands rather than have their deliveries performed by doctors. They still qualified for free postpartum care and the service of the foundling home.[19]

The post scriptum is shocking. The medical establishment's resistance to accepting Semmelweis's conclusions resulted in at least tens of thousands of preventable deaths. One among many other statistics indicates that at the famous La Maternité Hospital of Paris when puerperal fever raged between 1861 and 1864, almost one-fifth of all deliveries—I repeat, one out of five deliveries—resulted in the death of the mother.[20]

# 6

## EUGENICS, OYSTERS, SOUR SKIN, AND BREAST CANCER

WE ARE now reaching the end of the nineteenth century. The discovery of the microscopic agents of cholera, tuberculosis, puerperal fever, and pneumonia put an end to the debate about whether these feverish diseases were caused by miasms or germs. Medicine and public health were largely converted to the so-called germ theory of diseases advocated by the new scientific stars, Louis Pasteur and Robert Koch.

The availability of bacteriologic labs progressively tapered the need for group comparisons. Had Snow had access to bacteriological analyses of the water reaching the faucets of the two water companies' clients, he would not have needed to perform all the fieldwork he did to compare two large groups of Londoners. Had Semmelweis had access to a bacteriology lab, he could have compared the bacteriological content of the hands of doctors and midwives with that of the wombs of dying mothers to know that contaminated hands were the culprits. Whereas bacteriologists were uncovering one after the other the microbes responsible for the great fevers of the past, a surgeon, Joseph Lister, discovered the way to kill these microbes before they killed the patients. Asepsis and bacteriology had transformed the medical and public-health scene in a few decades. The hygiene of daily life in 1900 was considerably different from that of 1800.

Nevertheless, in many situations, questions could not be answered in labs. For example, labs could not deal with the long-term consequences of chronic infectious diseases, such as tuberculosis, or with situations in which contamination could not be traced to a unique source or, of course, when the disease did not have infectious origins.

In all these situations, group comparisons remained the only possible approach to assess treatment efficacy and modes of prevention. Solving these enigmas also required new keys. Epidemiologic methods had to be brought one step further and refined.

We will see in this chapter that the crude and naive mode of group comparisons that Snow, Louis, and Semmelweis applied would not suffice anymore to unravel scientific mysteries such as whether tuberculosis threatened the survival of the human species, what triggered typhoid and infant diarrhea,[1] or the causes of pellagra or cancer.

This troubled period, which comprised ten years of world war and a long world economic recession culminating in the Crash of 1929, witnessed the first implementation of the two principal designs of group comparisons still used today: the cohort study and the case–control study.

## RACIAL HYGIENE, TUBERCULOSIS, AND THE SURVIVAL OF THE HUMAN RACE

The combination of two of the most successful domains of science of the nineteenth century, Darwinian biology and bacteriology, produced a false and preposterous theory in the public-health circles of Europe and the United States around the early 1900s: eugenics.

The basic idea of eugenics was that the quality of a person depended on the quality of his or her genes. It falsely assumed that the laws of natural evolution also governed society. Eugenicists from across the full political spectrum believed that improvements in medical care and the growth of social legislation during the late nineteenth century had artificially altered the conditions of the natural struggle for survival within human societies. The new, milder social conditions allowed sick people, who in the past would have been severely disadvantaged, to survive and have progeny and therefore to taint the human race's genetic makeup.

Tuberculosis was emblematic of the eugenicists' fears. It was a very common disease. Around 1800, it regularly consumed the muscles and fat of the sick, who would ultimately die as a result of their steadily decreasing physical health. The word *consumption* was used interchangeably with

*phthisis* or *tuberculosis* to describe the disease. By 1900, the clinical picture of tuberculous patients had spectacularly changed. Many patients
who were better fed, lived in better homes, and sometimes isolated for
a period of time in more or less specialized centers called "sanatoriums"
survived. After their recovery, they apparently were able to live normal
lives and have families.

In Germany, eugenics was heralded by the Movement for Racial
Hygiene.[2] The Society for Racial Hygiene was created in 1905. Five years
later it had a branch in Stuttgart chaired by Wilhelm Weinberg, an MD
who in 1889 had opened a practice of general medicine and obstetrics.[3] In
1913, Weinberg published a book entitled *The Children of the Tuberculous*,[4]
describing the methods and results of a study involving 25,786 children
born from 7,098 parents from Stuttgart. This colossal study sought to
answer a central concern of racial hygienists: Did the children of tubercu-
losis-plagued parents survive longer than the children of nontuberculous
parents? If tuberculous had a survival advantage, then the genetic traits
among infected people would one day become dominant.

Imagine you live in Stuttgart, Germany, during 1913, and the ideas
underlying Weinberg's investigations seem less obnoxious than we know
them to be today. A reader unaware of the context, as I was when I first
read Weinberg's book, discovers the racial hygienic motivation only in its
last lines. *The Children of the Tuberculous* is an impressive scientific work
that initially does not seem driven by a dishonorable ideology.

Which population strategy would you propose to determine whether
the tuberculous had a survival advantage? The most logical suggestion,
given the historical context of the early 1900s, would be to draw a sample
of the population from Stuttgart and compare the mean age of two groups:
those who had been diagnosed with tuberculosis and those who had not.
But Weinberg noted that this approach would have been severely flawed.
The survey would have reached only the people who had lived long enough
to participate: What about those in the two groups who had already died?
The average age of the tuberculous could have appeared older if a minority of them, those that were extraordinarily resistant, survived to a very
old age and were reached by the survey, whereas the great majority died
very young and were missed. A typical nineteenth-century survey would
therefore not be functional.

Then what? How could Weinberg have designed a study that would discern the average age reached by tuberculous and nontuberculous people? How would you today measure the average longevity of an unselected group of people exposed to tuberculosis and compare it with that of an unselected group of people unexposed to tuberculosis? I am saying "today" in order for you not to be distracted by the fact that in 1913 all analyses were done with paper, pencil, and an indispensable eraser—no computer.

Weinberg's solution is mind-boggling. He identified all the people who had died from tuberculosis between 1873 and 1902 in the mortality registry of Stuttgart. He found 5,268 deaths. He also randomly selected a group of 1,830 people who had died during the same period of causes other than tuberculosis. He therefore had a total of 7,098 dead men and women. He then consulted the family registry of Stuttgart and documented all of their children. He found 25,786 of them. Back in the mortality registry, Weinberg recorded all the deaths that had occurred among these children up to the age of twenty. At the end of this Herculean task, Weinberg formed two cohorts: 18,212 children of tuberculous parents and 7,574 children of nontuberculous parents.

Weinberg found, as shown in figure 6.1, that 48 percent of the children with tuberculous parents died before age twenty. This proportion seems huge, right? One out of two children died before reaching age twenty. But 40 percent of the children in the nontuberculous group also died before reaching their twentieth birthday. That was the magnitude of perinatal and infant mortality experienced in Germany and other European countries at the time. Nevertheless, the study gave Weinberg an answer to his question: the children of the tuberculous lived a shorter life than those of the nontuberculous. Racial hygienic fears could be laid to rest: the survival advantage was on the side of the nontuberculous.[5]

Weinberg also established that tuberculous parents had fewer children than the nontuberculous. The data indicated that tuberculous parents had a smaller number of progeny because they died younger, not because they had a lower fertility. Weinberg therefore brought home that "from a racial hygienic perspective of the tuberculosis problem it is reassuring to note that the fertility of the tuberculous is not excessive and should remain far below that of the nontuberculous."[6]

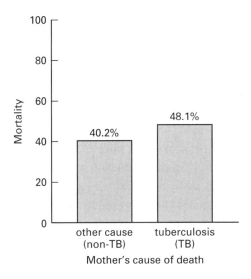

FIGURE 6.1  **Risk of Child's Death Before Age Twenty, Germany, c. 1900**

Risk of death before age twenty (as a percentage) of children of mothers who either died of tuberculosis (TB) or of another cause (non-TB) in Germany around 1900.

*Sources*: Weinberg 1913; see also Morabia 2007.

Weinberg also observed that longevity among the children of the tuberculous had a "strong social dependence." It followed a social gradient: children in the upper social classes were more likely to reach age twenty. Society could therefore control the impact of tuberculosis by improving the living conditions of the poor.

The lesson we can draw from Weinberg's remarkable endeavor is that besides population thinking and strategy, epidemiology requires rigorous study designs. For the first time in this book and also one of the first times in history, there is only one way to describe the group comparison made here. It unambiguously compared children exposed to tuberculosis at birth (because this was the cause of death of at least one of their parents) and children probably not exposed to tuberculosis (because their parents died from other causes.) The mortality risk before age twenty was 48 percent in the children of tuberculous parents versus 40 percent among the children of nontuberculous parents.

Weinberg himself died poor in 1937,[7] four years after Hitler came to power, and does not seem to have adhered to the Nazi ideology. The design of his study was novel. No one before him had performed such a long follow-up of such a large population. In epidemiology, a group of people followed up across time is now called a "cohort." Weinberg compared an "exposed" (tuberculous) cohort, comprising children whose parents had died of tuberculosis during specified time period, with an "unexposed" (nontuberculous) cohort. It was therefore a "cohort study."[8] We will come back to this type of study in the next chapter.

To the beliefs of racial hygiene, Weinberg opposed knowledge that is still valid today: tuberculosis has a "strong social dependence." Society can beneficially impact the survival of the human race by improving the living conditions of the poor, not by exterminating the poor.

## GUILTY OYSTERS, TYPHOID FEVER, AND THE INVENTION OF DIETARY QUESTIONNAIRES

Whether shellfish could transmit typhoid fever, a severe, often lethal bacterial infection of the gut, was a mystery in 1900. The English medical and lay press suspected that the fish trades laid oysters in sewage-contaminated areas. Animal food products were known to carry diseases such as tuberculosis and trichinosis. The typhoid-causing *Salmonella typhi* bacteria was discovered in 1886. But *Salmonella typhi* and oysters had still not been indisputably linked when an outbreak of typhoid fever made the news because it killed some important people.

On November 10, 1902, the local mayor of the old cathedral city of Winchester in the south of England organized a banquet at the city's Guildhall to celebrate the end of his term of office (figure 6.2). He invited past and present members of the city council, former mayors, doctors, lawyers, businessmen, members of the clergy, and other local notables.

The 134 guests sat along long tables and were served a series of exquisite dishes: clear (turtle) and thick soups, fish and seafood (oysters, turbot and lobster sauce, and smelts), roast beef, ham, tongue, kidneys, and sweetbread. They also had a choice of boiled or roasted mutton, poultry (capons, turkey), and game (venison, pheasants, partridge) with mushrooms and

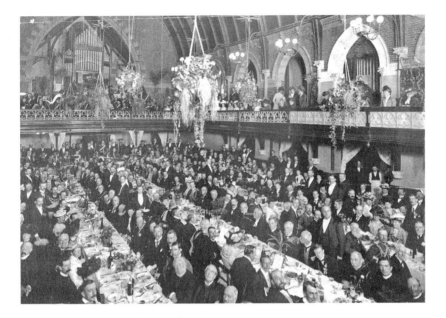

FIGURE 6.2

Winchester Guildhall Banquet in 1901, the year preceding the outbreak of enteric fever, showing the room where it started. It was customary in Britain at this period to hold banquets to celebrate the end of the local mayor's term of office. (Courtesy of Winchester Museums Service)

spinach. The rich desert buffet included red currant jelly, Sir Watkin Wynn pudding, charlotte russe, liqueur jellies, caramel cream, maraschino cream, meringues, and ice cream. Not to mention the cheese, salad, and aerated water available for the guests.

Shortly after the banquet, three of the guests died. Among them was Dr. William England, consultant surgeon to the Royal Hampshire County Hospital; the Reverend William Stephens, dean of Winchester Cathedral; and one (unnamed) waiter.

The story was widely reported in the national newspapers, and public alarm was palpable. It became evident that this episode was not isolated. Several cases of typhoid fever had also occurred in the area. The health authorities were pressed to go after the fishmongers.

The Local Government Board instructed a fine sleuth, Dr. H. Timbrell Bulstrode, a senior epidemiologist and a member of the London Epidemiologic Society, to find out. The facts were troubling enough: several cases of enteric fever (most likely typhoid fever) and many more of gastroenteritis of varying degrees of severity occurred among persons present at the banquet.[9]

Had Bulstrode asked for your advice on how to proceed with the investigation, what would you have said? It was one month after the banquet, the 134 guests had returned home, some were dead and others sick, and each one had probably consumed a different combination of dishes from the impressive number of items off the menu. It was too late to initiate some bacteriological analyses of the food. Would you have focused on the shellfish, the main suspects, even though there was no scientific evidence to incriminate them a priori?[10] Keep in mind that a host of other food products on the Winchester menu were also popularly associated with gastrointestinal disorders, such as turtle soup.

Taking a radically innovative approach, Bulstrode sent a copy of the menu to each of the guests. This was ingenious. Because the outbreak occurred at a banquet, there were good chances that all the potential sources of contamination were listed in the menu. Bulstrode asked each surviving guest (and proxies for those who died) to state which dishes they had consumed, whether they suffered any indisposition or illness shortly after the banquet, and, if so, the nature of such attacks and whether they ascribed them to the banquet.[11]

Bulstrode got an annotated menu back from all the guests or proxies, including for the dead waiter. This was a serious outbreak indeed: 46 percent of the 134 guests had fallen sick, 10 people (9 guests and a waiter) got enteric fever with severe diarrhea and a high temperature, and 40 percent (4 out of 10) of the enteric fever cases resulted in death.[12]

At this point, Bulstrode had two groups of people to consider: 63 people who had been more or less severely ill, including the 9 guests and a waiter who had had enteric fever, and 72 people who did not fall sick at all. This makes a total of 135 people. There was only one circumstance under which Bulstrode could solve the mystery by examining only the items consumed by the 63 sick attendees and therefore avoiding the paper-and-pencil analysis of the seventy-two other menus. Any clue?

Bulstrode's analysis could be simplified only if a single food item, consumed by all of the sick, had been responsible for the outbreak. Indeed, all but two of the sixty-three who had fallen more or less severely ill had eaten oysters. A deeper investigation of the two exceptions showed that their illnesses were unrelated to the banquet. Bulstrode eliminated turtle soup, the old copper vessel in which the soup had been prepared, and several other dishes from the list of suspects because many of the enteric fever cases had not eaten them.

Despite the tragic circumstances, Bulstrode had been lucky. The oysters, served raw, without further preparation in the kitchen, did not have the opportunity to contaminate the other foods. Had the culprit been a cook carrying *Salmonella typhi*, he would have contaminated multiple foods. People would have fallen sick after eating a variety of options, none of which being common to all the guests. In that case, the analysis of the sick persons' annotated menus would not have sufficed. Any idea about what Bulstrode should have done if many food items had been implicated in the outbreak?

Bulstrode would have had to compare the frequency of consumption of each of the food items on the menu between the sixty-three who got sick and the seventy-two who did not: the food items more frequently consumed by the sick than by those who did not suffer would have been deemed suspicious. Anne Hardy and I performed this group comparison: oysters stood out as the only food item much more frequently eaten by the sick.[13]

What was the impact of Bulstrode's report published many months later? It is hard to say. The results certainly received a significant amount of publicity in both popular and trade publications. Finally, the Worshipful Company of Fishmongers took steps in 1903 to ensure that shellfish from polluted layings did not reach the markets. Medical health officers across Britain became more vigilant regarding shellfish poisoning, and the public in general became cautious about eating shellfish.[14] Finding the guilty oyster is an epidemiologic achievement (Bulstrode did not rely on bacteriologic analyses): Bulstrode had devised an effective technique to measure the food consumed by 135 people, unknowingly initiating the long history of dietary questionnaires.

## POOR DIET, MENTAL DISORDER,
## AND (ALMOST) THE NOBEL PRIZE

"Miasms are the source of all diseases" was the rule behind the popular beliefs of the nineteenth century. When this rule lost its credibility, it was quickly replaced by a new tenet that posited that "germs are the source of all diseases." One after the other, the microscopic agents of anthrax, tuberculosis, cholera, typhoid, puerperal fever, pneumonia, and so on were being identified. Thus, in 1907 when the United States witnessed an epidemic of a loathsome skin disease called pellagra, which was often associated with dementia, it was initially attributed to a still unidentified germ. A privately funded house-to-house survey of pellagra cases in the cotton mill districts of South Carolina had concluded that pellagra was most likely an infectious disease caused by a still unknown agent.[15]

Until 1907, pellagra had been rare in the United States, but not among the European peasantry, in which it had been described since 1735, particularly in agricultural areas where the manpower was chronically malnourished. Often mistaken for leprosy because of the thickening and abundant desquamation of the skin, it had been dubbed disease of the "sour skin," which is what the Italian term *pelle agra* means. Its four unique cardinal symptoms began with a *d*: dermatitis, diarrhea, dementia, and death.

The epidemic that burst out in 1907 in the American South was massive. By 1912, 25,000 cases, called "pellagrins," had been diagnosed in state asylums and communities. Forty-three percent of cases died of their disease. This formidable growth of pellagra was not confined to the southern states. The US Congress asked the Surgeon General to investigate the disease. In 1914, the surgeon assigned Joseph Goldberger (figure 6.3), then a medical officer in the US Public Health Service, to investigate what was "undoubtedly one of the knottiest and most urgent problems facing the Service at the present time."[16]

After less than three months of field investigation, Goldberger was convinced that pellagra was not communicable. He observed that nurses or attendants of pellagra patients were themselves always free of the disease.[17] In mental hospitals and orphanages, the disease hit inmates, but never staff. Well-to-do people seemed immune to the condition. Goldberger believed that an infectious disease could not neatly differentiate between

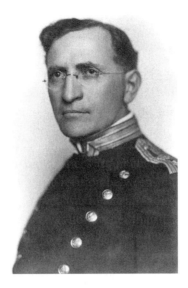

FIGURE 6.3

Joseph Goldberger. (From Wikimedia Commons)

inmates and employees or between rich and poor. He favored the hypothesis that a superior diet, rich in "vitamins," protected people from pellagra. But he needed to prove it.

Step by step, Goldberger built a case about the dietary nature of pellagra. He began by showing that more lean meat and lentils in the diet of two orphanages in Jackson, Mississippi, prevented the recurrence of pellagra. Generally about half of the children at the orphanages between ages six and twelve suffered annually from pellagra. Throughout the twelve months during which Goldberger improved their diets, not a single case occurred. Goldberger obtained similar results in a psychiatric asylum in Georgia.

Goldberger was aware that simply by changing the diet of all the inmates, he could not defend his hypothesis against the criticism of those who would say that he had just been lucky in doing so during a year without any pellagra cases. He noted that "the ideal for the experiment would have been, of course, to retain for purpose of comparison, a control group at each of the institutions."[18] He wanted to modify the diet of only half of the inmates. But this was not feasible. The poor public institutions were not equipped to prepare and serve two different meals. Goldberger was nonetheless convinced that pellagra could be entirely eliminated through the diet and that it was not a communicable disease.

Goldberger decided to show that he could incite pellagra among healthy volunteers by submitting them to a diet poor in protein-rich food. It would be unthinkable to conduct such an unethical study today: participants can die from the disease. Goldberger obtained the authorization to produce pellagra by means of a typical poor southern corn-based diet among healthy volunteer convicts of the Mississippi State Penitentiary. In 1915, six of the eleven volunteer convicts developed typical signs of pellagra and were in pain for months. They were in exchange (with one exception) relieved of their ball and chain. In contrast, there were no cases of pellagra among the comparison, a group of thirty-five convicts who had been under observation for the same duration of time but whose diet had not been modified.

At that point, in 1916, Goldberger designed experiments to demonstrate that pellagra could not be transmitted from humans to humans. In so-called filth parties, he injected blood from patients with pellagra into the shoulder muscles of sixteen healthy volunteers, including himself and his wife. He also mixed extracts of skin parings, nasal secretions, urine, and feces from patients with pellagra into a wheat dough concoction that was swallowed by all volunteers. These "filth party" experiments were repeated seven times. Although many participants developed diarrhea and nausea, no signs of pellagra were ever noted.

## The Cotton Mill Study

In order to be completely convincing, Goldberger needed to demonstrate that the recurring pellagra outbreaks occurred among malnourished families. He needed to move from clinical studies and experiments that were restricted to selected populations to a real-life test of his hypothesis. He turned to the cotton mill villages, which were badly affected by pellagra every summer.

This research proved to be quite a challenge. How would you have proceeded? To design the appropriate study, you need to know that the history of pellagra in the United States is closely related to that of the cotton industry.

After the abolition of slavery, tenant farming was used to maintain southern agriculture. Sharecroppers were assigned parcels of land to grow the landowners' cotton and jointly guarantee their own subsistence. The typical sharecropper's lot was a dilapidated cabin, a few corn plants, and a luxurious but inedible growth of cotton. In order to maximize their potential income, the tenants planted as much cotton as they could and ignored their own nutritional needs, which could have been supplied with a vegetable garden and some chickens.

The cotton was then brought to mills, where it was transformed into yarn and fabric by similarly exploited workers. These poor workers and their families subsisted from April to September mostly on what they bought in the landowners' stores, a diet made of cornbread, fatback, and black molasses, in which the corn meal was the only source of protein. Many villages paid in trade checks that could only be redeemed at the mill's store. Sharecroppers, whose fields surrounded the mill, had no fresh meat or milk to sell. In some villages, however, workers were paid in cash and had access to local farmers' markets.

Goldberger chose to study cotton mills in the vicinity of Spartanburg, South Carolina. The cotton workers and their families were both poor and malnourished. The challenge Goldberger faced (and now you do too) was to separate poverty from malnourishment in order to demonstrate which variable was the immediate cause of pellagra.

Thus, how would you have proceeded to identify the cause of pellagra in these mill villages? You likely opt for some form of a group comparison of pellagra incidence between cotton worker families based on income or diet quality. Goldberger did too. Edgar Sydenstricker, an economist and statistician familiar with population data, and his assistant George A. Wheeler joined him on this project. Together, in the spring of 1916, they designed and conducted a methodologically remarkable investigation.[19]

They selected seven cotton mill villages, enumerated their populations, and sampled 750 households, comprising a total of 4,160 mill workers and their families, exclusively of white, Anglo-Saxon origin. Apparently, very few African Americans were employed in the industrial processing of the cotton. To visualize the type of challenges that Goldberger and

Sydenstricker faced, consider how you would have measured income, diet, and pellagra incidence among mostly illiterate people.

From the company books and interviews, Goldberger and Sydenstricker computed an average income per family based on the number of household members and the adult/children composition.[20] The assessment of the household diet consisted of detailed information provided by the household members, by farmers and travelling food peddlers, and by the factory shops. It was performed between April 16 and June 15, before the expected, sharp seasonal rise in pellagra incidence. In addition, twice per week the study personnel visited all the houses and counted the new cases of pellagra indicated by clearly defined skin lesions that were symmetrically distributed on their bodies.

Fortunately for the investigators, the variation in income and diet among the sharecropper families was sufficient to perform a meaningful comparison. The study showed that very poor families ate more salted pork and corn, similar amounts of dry beans, but less green vegetables, fresh fruits, and meat than the better-off families. Pellagra was more common among the poorer families. That was the first significant result. In this group comparison of households with different income levels, real risks of developing pellagra over the summer differed drastically between the poorest households, with 42.7 cases per 1,000 individuals, and the highest-income households, with 3.4 cases per 1,000, a twelve-fold difference. Risks for the intermediate income groups lay between these two extremes.

Thus, income was associated with pellagra, but was it because of insufficient vegetable and animal food or because of another factor associated with poverty and therefore with susceptibility to infection that subjected the poor households to pellagra more often? A gigantic research effort ended in scientific stalemate: Was it diet or infection? The key question that motivated the whole endeavor remained unanswered. Comparing poorer with better-off households was equivalent to comparing households consuming essentially corn meal and grits with households that had access to milk and fresh products. What to do? You could say, like Jagger and Richard, "Yeah, I really don't know," but Goldberger and Sydenstricker devised a superb solution, a strategy that no one had seemingly used before.

They compared the diets of two villages (out of the seven studied) with the most extreme risks of pellagra: 0 per 1,000 in Newry and 64.6 per

1,000 in Inman Mills. Both villages were poor, but in the pellagrous Inman Mills income was higher than in the nonpellagrous Newry. Poverty could therefore not explain the differences in pellagra risk between Inman Mills and Newry.

In the nonpellagrous village of Newry, 58.1 percent of the households reported having purchased fresh meat twice or more in two weeks, whereas this proportion was only 8.5 percent in the pellagrous village of Inman Mills.

As shown in figure 6.4, the dietary contrast was even stronger for the combined consumption of milk, butter, eggs, fresh vegetables and fruits, and poultry: 83.3 percent of the Newry households consumed

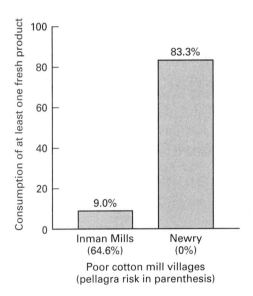

FIGURE 6.4 **Consumption of Fresh Food Products and Incidence of Pellagra, South Carolina, 1916**

Comparison of the proportion of poor households consuming fresh food (milk, butter, eggs, vegetables, fruit, poultry) over a two-week period, May 16–30, 1916, and the incidence of pellagra in two cotton mill villages of South Carolina. The two villages were among the poorest of the study. There were no cases of pellagra in Newry, and the highest risk of pellagra among the seven villages studied was observed in Inman Mills.

*Source*: Goldberger 1920.

these products in the spring when the dietary assessment had been performed, as opposed to only 9 percent of the households in Inman Mills. The late medical historian Harry Marks described the reasons for these differences in fresh-food consumption: "Newry, the non-pellagra village in Oconee County, was ideally situated in a region of diversified farming. A village market sold fresh meat throughout the year, and the district's extensive truck farming kept the same market well-supplied with vegetables. By contrast, a second village, Inman Mills, in Spartan-burg County, offered no local alternative to the company store. More importantly, it was situated in a cotton-dominated region, with few farmers growing vegetables or raising livestock to sell in town. These circumstances left Inman Mills' villagers poorly supplied with fresh vegetables, milk, or meat."[21]

Was this a group comparison? Yes, even though it was unusual in the sense that it aggregated people at the village level as opposed to at the household level, as in the previous analyses. The comparison was between a village with a high rate of pellagra and a village with no pellagra. It was found that one village had a better diet. But in the context this additional information indicated that poor people developed pellagra because they were deprived of milk, meat, and fresh products. This original, "multilevel" approach therefore enabled Goldberger to separate the effect of income from that of diet.

### Missed Nobel Prize

Goldberger finally amassed conclusive evidence to validate his position that improving access to fresh food for the poor was the way to stop the epidemic of pellagra and prevent its recurrence.[22] After disputing the belief that pellagra was an infectious disease, Goldberger convincingly defended the theory that it was a nutritional disease caused by a lack of a still unidentified vitamin that he called the "pellagra preventive" factor and that many scientists proceeded to call the "G factor," where G stood for "Goldberger."

We know today that pellagra attacks the skin, the guts, and the brain because of a deficiency of the B3 vitamin niacin, which plays an indispens-able role in cell metabolism. By definition, vitamins are molecules that the human body cannot synthesize. The body's synthesis of niacin depends on the availability of the essential amino acid, tryptophan, which abounds in milk, cheese, fish, meat, and eggs. The absence of niacin impairs the fast reproductive cycle of skin cells, inducing the leperlike lesions, and causes dementia and diarrhea by blocking the synthesis of serotonin, a hormone regulating intestinal activity and many cerebral functions. But why had the United States South lacked niacin for thirty years? The epidemic started suddenly in 1907, had one peak during World War I, and had the second peak during the Great Depression of 1929–1933. Yet by 1940 the disease had disappeared.

The abrupt start of the epidemic coincided with the introduction of a new method of milling corn around 1900. This technological change removed the "germ" or embryo in the corn kernel and stripped the corn of the majority of its nutriments.[23] In a nutshell, mill workers, sharecroppers, and their families were forced to live on a corn-based diet in order to get income out of their fields or industrial work, but corn had become less nutritious than it was in the past, unbeknownst to them.

The epidemic recess coincided with the food industry's tendency after 1941 to fortify food with amino acids and vitamins, thus artificially reintroducing them into the corn meal. Moreover, after the Great Depression, southern farmers diverted from cotton. The new crops—soybeans, peanuts, peas, citrus, and other fruits or garden vegetables—could, unlike cotton, also feed the workers. By the end of the 1920s, there was a general consensus that Goldberger had been right since 1914. It is the kind of brilliant prediction that qualifies a scientist for the Nobel Prize. When in 1929 the Nobel Committee decided to dedicate its prize to the discoverers of disease-causing vitamin deficiencies, Goldberger was a potential laureate. Unfortunately, he died in January of that same year and could not be among the winners.[24]

## WOMAN, WOMEN, AND BREAST CANCER

In this chapter enters the first woman (in this book at least) to have contributed to the evolution of group comparisons. When Janet Lane-Claypon (figure 6.5) rises as a pioneer of epidemiology, women's role in society

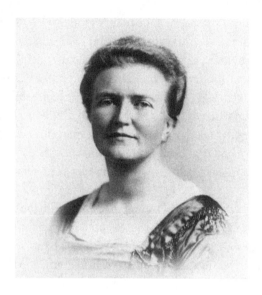

FIGURE 6.5

Janet Lane-Claypon. Photo by Stereoscopic Co., London. (From Images from the History of Medicine, National Library of Medicine, Washington, DC)

and in science is rapidly evolving. Women are recognized in science, literature, and politics. Marie Curie received Nobel Prizes in physics (1903) and chemistry (1911). Selma Lagerloef received a Nobel Prize in Literature (1909). The Polish-born Rosa Luxemburg was a prominent of the German Social-Democratic Party until 1919. To name a few.

Lane-Claypon had an outstanding career. She was the first woman ever to receive a research scholarship from the British Medical Society. In a group portrait of twenty-four members, researchers, and fellows of the Lister Institute of Preventative Medicine in 1907, Lane-Claypon is one of the only two women pictured. After graduating as a doctor in 1910, she rapidly moved to public health. She was a medical inspector and then dean of the London School of Medicine for Women until in 1923 she joined the civil service and was trusted with a series of research tasks about breast cancer, a disease that had newly attracted considerable interest in the Ministry of Health.

## Breast Cancer and Lactation

Toward the end of the nineteenth century, breast cancer was believed to be a "constitutional disease," hereditary and incurable. Surgically removing the tumor was deemed useless. But pathologists linked breast cancer to degenerative changes in the cells of the mammary gland, and the progress of surgery—in particular aseptic techniques, anesthesia, and mastectomies raised the hope that an early operation could cure breast cancer.

However, in 1923 the Committee on Cancer reporting to Minister of Health Neville Chamberlain noted that too few women looked for surgical advice and treatment at an early stage of the disease. Was it because of all the "opinions and beliefs" that predisposed women were doomed to die from their disease? Another "belief, fairly generally entertained" was that "improper lactation" was a predisposing cause of cancer of the breast. The committee therefore asked Lane-Claypon to determine whether breastfeeding "for too long or for too short a period" could cause breast cancer using an approach that would be more valid than "any attempts based only on existing records or on the collection of opinions."[25]

In this context, how would you have proceeded to determine whether duration of breastfeeding was related to breast cancer? A logical answer would be to identify a cohort of women having breastfed all their children for a "short" period and a comparable cohort of women having breastfed at least one child for a "long" period. All women would be free of cancer when entering the study. Then the number of new breast cancer cases diagnosed in each group would be counted over some period of time. If more cases occurred in one of the two cohorts, you would be able to conclude that breastfeeding was related to breast cancer.

In theory, this approach was correct. In practice, it would have required the follow-up of very large groups of women. The rate of breast cancer in the United Kingdom was about 20 per 100,000 per year in 1925. Lane-Claypon would have had to follow 100,000 people for five years to accrue at least 100 cases of breast cancer in her study. Designing such a large-scale study in order to investigate an association that was still hypothetical would not have been reasonable.

Would you have an alternative suggestion? Consider modifying the question. Instead of asking whether breastfeeding is related to breast cancer, ask whether people who got breast cancer have breastfed for a "long" period as often as people who did not get breast cancer. For example, if long durations of breastfeeding protected from breast cancer, then women who developed breast cancer must be less likely to have breastfed for twelve months or more than their counterpart who remained free of breast cancer, right? And vice versa if breastfeeding were deleterious.

Comparing the breastfeeding history of people with and without breast cancer had a huge practical advantage, then. Hospitals concentrated breast cancer cases among populations of several million adults. At hospitals, hundreds of cases of breast cancer could be recruited in relatively short amounts of time. Moreover, they could be compared with patients admitted for other diseases during the same period of time. This "hospital-based case–control study" was a cost- and time-effective strategy when studying a disease as rare as breast cancer.

That was Lane-Claypon's choice. A small number of trained persons, including her, would interview hundreds of women admitted to hospitals for breast cancer about all the so-called predisposing factors and do the same thing with a same number of women apparently free of breast cancer, but whose conditions of life were broadly comparable to those of the cancer cases. The study took place in 1924 in hospitals of London and Glasgow, two populous centers.

Was it a group comparison? Yes, Lane-Claypon compared 508 cases of cancer of the breast with 509 controls. Both groups had, on average, similar nationality, age (most of the women were older than forty-five), marital status, occupation, and number of deceased children (used as an indicator of social class). Of all the episodes of the evolution of epidemiology reviewed in this book, this is the first group comparison that can undoubtedly be characterized as a "case–control" study.

All mothers readily remembered the duration of lactation for each of their children even if they had had many. Among the married women, 24.1 percent of the 261 cases and 42.1 percent of the 280 controls had had more than five children. In itself, this finding suggested that multiple pregnancies could protect against breast cancer. The results for breastfeeding were also reassuring: 19.8 percent of the 868 children of 200 of the married

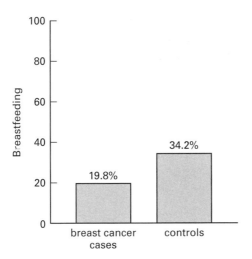

FIGURE 6.6 **Breastfeeding for Twelve Months or More by Children of Women with and Without Breast Cancer, London and Glasgow, c. 1880–1924**

Case–control study comparing the proportions of the 868 children of 200 married breast cancer cases and of the 1,337 children of 280 married controls who were breastfed for twelve months or more.

*Source*: Lane-Claypon 1926.

breast cancer cases had been breastfed for twelve months or more versus 34.2 percent of the 1,337 children of the 280 married controls (figure 6.6). Lane-Claypon could have concluded that breastfeeding protected against breast cancer. This was, however, a bold inference to draw from single study. Instead, in a minimalistic statement, she stressed that the beliefs about breastfeeding's predisposition to cancer could be safely abandoned: "that lactation for any period from 6 months to 2 years cannot be shown to have any detrimental effect on the breast in relation to the later development of cancer."[26]

In her remarkable report, Lane-Claypon debunked many of the old beliefs about predisposing factors. Her findings that fewer children, an older age at first birth, and a shorter duration of lactation increase the risk of breast cancer are still current knowledge.[27]

Lane-Claypon's innovative case–control study alone would have sufficed to admit her to the pantheon of great epidemiologists. Her work, however, enriched the methods of epidemiology in many other domains.[28] Her sudden retirement in 1929, when at the age of fifty-two she married Sir Edward Forber, was therefore baffling. Or perhaps not so baffling: the English civil service did not allow women to work after marriage. She terminated her career, moved to the countryside, and lived forty more years quietly with her husband until her death in 1967. She was ninety.

# 7

# TOBACCO AND HEALTH

## The Great Controversy

TWENTIETH-CENTURY POPULATIONS demonstrated a formidable attraction to tobacco and its smoke—an aggressively marketed, addictive product.[1] In just a few decades, a substantial fraction of the working population began to smoke tobacco in the form of a cigarette.

How could cigarette smoking, a rare habit in 1900, become ubiquitous by 1950? Psychologists emphasize the strong addictive properties of nicotine. Economists point to cigarettes' affordability made possible by industrial production. Toxicologists note that cigarettes are an ideal way to titrate the blood concentration of nicotine. Sociologists mention the effects on cigarette sales of an aggressive marketing policy oriented toward all sectors of society—men, women, and children.[2] But the mass consumption of cigarettes also took off during a time marked by profound change in the Western way of life. Physical activity, humans' main source of antistress sedation, was rapidly replaced in the daily routine by mechanical transportation and home appliances. Tobacco may thus have also served as a sedative.

## CIGARETTES, THORACIC SURGERY, AND "PACKAGES OF REST"

When the cigarette became a product of mass consumption, smokers experienced positive effects. In particular, they said it helped them to relax and concentrate.

A 1936 *Scientific American* editorial underscored that the psychotropic effect of tobacco was the main reason why smokers loved their addiction: "The most interesting effects of smoking are those which occur to the central nervous system. Like alcohol, tobacco is often called a 'stimulant'—it is said to pep you up—but instead, much like alcohol, it is mainly the opposite: a sedative. Professor Mendenhall points out that it has an effect similar to that of rest, and he called cigarettes 'a package of rest.' This is probably the main basis of the smoking habits although in many cases the 'feel' of the cigarette or pipe or cigar in the mouth is the basis of the same habit, on its own account. The source of the 'rest' in tobacco is the nicotine in it."[3]

This editorial considered sedation to be the "most" interesting effect of smoking. Because rest is generally good for health, the overall idea was that smoking was a healthy habit. The tobacco industry built its marketing strategy on such beliefs and even involved doctors. "More doctors smoke Camel than any other brand of cigarette" was the motto of an advertising campaign. Many doctors indeed had a positive attitude toward cigarettes: a 1945 American Medical Association poster illustrated medical progress by showing a man able to light up his cigarette using a prosthetic arm.

Meanwhile, there was cause for concern. Closely following the rise of cigarette consumption, mortality from lung cancer increased rapidly worldwide. The phenomenon was immediately apparent because the disease was lethal in almost all cases, death typically occurring within one year of diagnosis. Between 1922 and 1947, the annual number of deaths from lung cancer increased roughly fifteen times in the United Kingdom. In the United States, crude death rates from lung cancer had climbed from 3.1 per 100,000 men in 1930 to 19.8 in 1950. Death rates were also rising in Switzerland, Denmark, Canada, Australia, Turkey, and Japan. This increasing number of deaths from cancer of the lung was one of the most striking changes in the pattern of mortality.

Opinions diverged about how to interpret the magnitude of this new phenomenon. Some denied that lung cancer was occurring more frequently. Instead, they attributed the rise in mortality to improved diagnosis from the new, widespread use of chest X-rays. Others proposed that it was a consequence of an aging society: people lived longer and therefore died from cancer more often. Others incriminated air pollution or the flu—some saw the lung cancer epidemic as a sequel to the 1918 Great Influenza Epidemic.

Nonetheless, before 1950, several scientists claimed that tobacco caused cancer. Tobacco, essentially a habit among men, provided a better explanation for the fact that lung cancer killed five to ten times more men than women than did air pollution or the flu. I have listed these claims here. What do you think was the common weakness in the evidence that supported them?

1. In the late 1920s, Angel Honorio Roffo, director of a cancer institute in Buenos Aires, produced skin tumors after applying tarry residue from distilled tobacco smoke to the ear lining of rabbits.[4] In several articles, he speculated that tobacco caused lung cancer in humans, too.

2. By the 1930s, pathologists, surgeons, and vital statisticians had noticed and documented the increased frequency of lung cancer.

3. In 1938, the statistician Raymond Pearl at the Johns Hopkins School of Hygiene and Public Health in Baltimore showed that tobacco reduced the life expectancy of heavy smokers by about ten years compared to that of never smokers.[5]

4. In 1939, Alton Ochsner and Michael DeBakey, thoracic surgeons from New Orleans, were able to report on eighty-six lung cancer patients who were treated by surgical removal of a lung. This was a large descriptive series for a disease that was extremely rare in 1900. They insisted that "in [their] opinion the increase of smoking with the universal custom of inhaling is probably a responsible factor as the inhaled smoke, constantly repeated over a long period of time undoubtedly is a source of chronic irritation of the bronchial mucosa."[6] They did not mention whether each of the eighty-six cases, which they described one by one, smoked.

Wasn't this quite an impressive set of discordant voices, all pointing to the harmful health effects of tobacco? Why is it that they were not heard? Well, Roffo's animal studies could not be simply extrapolated to humans. Pearl was on the right track, but he had studied overall longevity, not cancer. In contrast to Jane Lane-Claypon (see chapter 6), Ochsner and DeBakey never used a comparison group consisting of people free of lung cancer but of the same age, gender, and ethnicity as the diseased group in order to reveal whether they had similar smoking habits or not. The common weakness of all these opinions was that they were not derived from rigorous group comparisons in a human population relating tobacco use to a cause of death, in particular lung cancer.

## PRE-1945 COMPARATIVE STUDIES OF TOBACCO AND LUNG CANCER

Three pre-1950 studies did indeed compare the smoking habits of people with lung cancer and of people without lung cancer, but they were not very convincing either. In 1931, Frederick Hoffman, head of the San Francisco Cancer Survey and an experienced epidemiologist, provided early comparative evidence that smoking could cause lung cancer. Hoffman, through interviews, found 46 percent of "heavy smokers" among all patients diagnosed with cancer, but 67 percent among patients diagnosed with lung cancer specifically. In comparison, only 12.5 percent of a group of industrial workers were heavy smokers. Hoffman concluded that "smoking habits unquestionably increase[d] the liability to cancer of the mouth, throat, esophagus, larynx and lungs." He added that "the increase in cancer of the lung [was] . . . traceable to cigarette smoking and inhalation of cigarette smoke." He also evoked the harmful effect of passive smoking: "The gross amount of air pollution as the result of almost universal smoking habits . . . applies to the development of cancer of the lungs which occur among women . . . frequently among those who are not smokers."[7]

Two studies comparing patients who died from lung cancer with groups of subjects free of lung cancer were published in Germany in 1939 and 1943 by card-carrying members of the Nazi Party.[8] The studies had strikingly similar characteristics and weaknesses. Indeed, the authors of the second study claimed to have attempted to reproduce the findings of the first study.

In 1939, Franz Mueller compared the smoking habits of lung cancer patients with those of undefined "healthy" men. And in 1943, Eberhard Schairer and Erich Schoeniger compared the smoking habits of lung cancer patients, patients with other cancers, and a group of also undefined "normal" men. Both studies found a larger proportion of heavy smokers among the men with lung cancer than among the controls and concluded that tobacco caused lung cancer. However, the 1943 study failed to say how they classified and analyzed pipe smokers even though in the 1930s pipe smoking was common among older smokers.

The main problem of the studies by Mueller and by Schairer and Schoeniger was the puzzling lack of information about the men free of lung cancer who provided the referent smoking habits in the population. Mueller wrote that they were healthy and the same age. Schairer and Schoeniger mentioned that they were fifty-three- and fifty-four-year-old men from Jena. The dissertation Schoeniger wrote on the basis of the second study is also silent about the identification, recruitment, and characteristics of the live subjects—other than the information provided in his and Schairer's publication. The paucity of information about the control group distinguishes these two studies from all the case–control studies performed before 1945 that I am aware of, including the study by Janet Lane-Claypon discussed in chapter 6. It was obvious to American and English authors who also studied chronic diseases such as cancer (but not lung cancer) and heart diseases that the validity of the comparisons relied on the selection of the controls. These authors therefore took great pain to describe the selection process of the control group and to tabulate their age, gender, and other relevant characteristics.[9] They gave sufficient detail about the method they used for us to closely repeat what they did if we wished to. In contrast, the selection of the controls in the two German studies is mysterious.

The best that can be said about the studies emanating from the Nazi period is that they were amateurish. They did not break new ground and were not qualitatively better than that performed, as we have seen, by Hoffman before them in the United States.

Altogether, the pre-1945 studies of smoking and lung cancer were too weak to uncover the link between cigarette smoking and lung cancer. There are two telling testimonials of the cigarette's ability to fool scientists and doctors for almost half of century. A 1932 editorial by *The Lancet* summarized the feeling in the scientific community that the dire health effects of exposure to tobacco smoke still had to be demonstrated: "However difficult it may be to prove the case against cigarette-smoking, it has not yet been cleared from suspicion."[10] The second testimony is by Dr. Charles S. Cameron for *Time* magazine, reporting his impression of a March 1949 conference of the American Cancer Society and the National Cancer Institute in Memphis: "For every expert who blames tobacco for cancer of the lung, there is another expert who says tobacco is not the cause."[11]

By 1949, many still believed that cigarettes were "packages of rest," and there were no rigorous group comparisons to contradict them. Convincing proofs that tobacco smoke was the most important cause of lung cancer were soon to be provided, however, by several studies comparing the smoking habits of a group of lung cancer cases to those of a group of controls free of lung cancer.

These studies began to be published in 1950. This is also a watershed year for the change in opinion about lung cancer trends in two of the most influential and respected British medical journals. In 1942, there were still doubts that the rising trend in cancer of the lung observed in recent years was real.[12] But in 1952 *The Lancet* editorialized that few trends were more dramatic than the rise in the notified deaths from cancer of the lung during the previous thirty years and that there was thus "little doubt" that the increase was both real and numerically important.[13]

## THE NAIVE APPROACH TO
## SMOKING AND LUNG CANCER

Each time I see a movie of the mid–twentieth century, taking place anywhere in Europe or in North America, I am struck by the fact that nearly everybody smokes and does so almost constantly throughout the movie. Aren't you? Smokers and nonsmokers alike inhaled the scrolls of tobacco smoke all day long at home, at work, in buses, on planes and trains, and in subways. Doctors smoked in front of their patients and teachers in front of their students. The ambient air of bars and restaurants was constantly filled with tobacco smoke.

It may seem obvious today that smoking tobacco was responsible for the epidemic of lung cancer that began around 1910 and rose unabated until about 1960 in most Western countries. However, for those who believed lung cancer had environmental causes, there was another plausible candidate just as ubiquitous as cigarettes, but more smelly than tobacco: the dramatic increase in car usage and its related infrastructure (e.g., tarred roads and bridges). In some ways, cars were a clean mode of transportation in comparison to horses that had covered the nineteenth-century roads with manure. At the same time, cars filled the air with the stinking exhaust of combustion engines and dust that emanated from the tarring of the roadways and bridges. Another environmental candidate besides tar dust was air pollution from gasworks, industrial plants, and coal fires, which also offensively filled the atmosphere of modern societies.

Studying lung cancer in 1945 presented the same type of methodologic challenges as when Lane-Claypon had studied breast cancer twenty years earlier: the disease was rare in the population, but most cases were admitted in hospitals at a later point in their development. Comparing cases and controls in hospitals was the most cost- and time-effective strategy. Of the several case–control studies of lung cancer published after 1945, I discuss three here that had novel methodologic features. It is clear from the introductions in the papers reporting the results of these studies that at their inception their authors did not consider the association between tobacco and lung cancer as having been established.

Morton L. Levin and his colleagues at the New York State Department of Health performed their study at Roswell Park Memorial Institute in Buffalo, a laboratory and hospital devoted solely to the study of cancer.[14] This institution had the particularity of interviewing about their smoking habits all patients on the day of admission, before they underwent any diagnostic work. Levin and his colleagues had therefore an opportunity to control for an important source of concern about the smoking history information obtained from patients with lung cancer and controls: Could being diagnosed with lung cancer affect the way study participants answered the questions about their past smoking experiences? Would the discovery of a tumor in the lung prompt the patients to report more exposure than they would have reported had they not develop the disease? This potential source of bias would be less prominent at the Roswell Park Memorial Institute because patients were interviewed about their smoking habits upon admission, *before* a diagnosis of lung cancer had been established or ruled out.

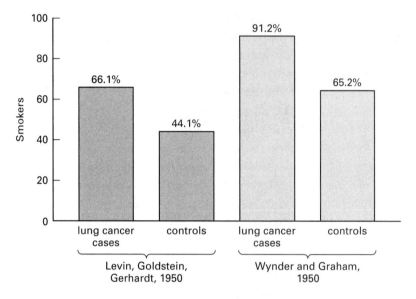

FIGURE 7.1 **Cigarette Smokers as a Percentage of Lung Cancer Cases and Controls Free of Lung Cancer, Late 1940s**

Two North American case–control studies comparing the proportion of cigarette smokers among men having lung cancer (the cases) with a group of men admitted for diseases other than cancer (the controls). Both studies were published in the same issue of the *Journal of the American Medical Association*.

*Sources*: Levin, Goldstein, and Gerhardt 1950; Wynder and Graham 1950.

Approximately half the patients admitted to the institute with a suspicion of cancer were subsequently found to have some cancer. They could serve as cases, whereas those with symptoms at the same sites that proved not to be due to cancer could serve as a source of comparable controls. Between 1938 and 1948, 236 men were discharged with a diagnosis of lung cancer. These lung cancer cases were compared with a group of 605 noncancer controls. The proportion of cigarette smokers was 66.1 percent among the lung cancer cases and 44.1 percent among the noncancer controls (figure 7.1, *left*). Age could not explain these differences. The conclusion read, "[T]he data suggest, although they do not establish, a causal relation between cigarette smoking and cancer of the lung."[15]

The second study was remarkable for its magnitude: it included 605 men with lung cancer from several hospitals and private practices around the United States and another 780 men admitted to general hospitals without cancer of the lung who served as controls. It was conducted in 1948 and 1949 by Ernst L. Wynder while he was still a medical student and Professor Evarts A. Graham, renowned thoracic surgeon and chairman of the Department of Surgery at Washington University School of Medicine in St. Louis. To boost the homogeneity of the case group, the study was limited to epidermoid cancer, usually occurring in large airways directly impacted by tobacco smoke. The case–control comparisons were made within homogeneous age categories. Among the men, the proportions of cigarette smokers were 91.2 percent among the lung cancer cases and 65.2 percent among the controls (figure 7.1, *right*). One out of two lung cancer cases was an excessive or chain smoker compared to one out of five controls without cancer. Wynder and Graham's paper concluded that "excessive and prolonged use of tobacco, especially cigarets [*sic*], seems to be an important factor in the induction of bronchogenic carcinoma."[16]

The design and results of these two studies were different from anything that had been produced before in studying lung cancer.

Both compared a group of patients who had lung cancer (the "cases") with a clearly identified group of hospital patients free of lung cancer (the "controls"). This way of designing group comparisons is what we now call a "case–control study." In 1950, it was called a "retrospective study" because it selected the compared groups on the basis of the presence or absence of the studied disease and inquired retrospectively about past exposure to the incriminated cause.

How much health harm was observed? None of the studies could directly answer this question. Both observed more cigarette smokers among the cases than among the controls: 66 percent versus 44 percent for Levin and 91 percent versus 65 percent for Wynder. Differences in the amount that the cases smoked were even more extreme.

Nevertheless, these results were not substantial enough to convince a skeptical mind. The two studies pointed in the same direction: lung cancer cases had smoked more cigarettes in the past than had the controls, and so an association between the two was drawn. But the studies did not directly answer the causal question: Does cigarette smoking cause lung cancer?

LUNG CANCER → (associated with) PAST CIGARETTE SMOKING

CIGARETTE SMOKING → (causes) LUNG CANCER

These two studies were naive in the sense that their authors reported only case–control differences in smoking frequency. They did not seem to perceive that because of the close connection between the two questions, they could have expressed their results in terms of how much harm smoking tobacco incurred. Do you see how this could have been done? One of the possible answers is given in the next section.

## THE INGENIOUS APPROACH TO STUDYING SMOKING AND LUNG CANCER

In 1948, the chief of the Medical Research Council (the English equivalent of the National Institutes of Health in the United States) commissioned Austin Bradford Hill to conduct a study about the causes of lung cancer.[17] Hill was a highly respected epidemiologist, a pioneer of randomized clinical trials, author of a textbook of medical statistics, and professor of "medical statistics." He hired Richard Doll, a research assistant at the time, to run the study.

At first glance, the design of an English study of tobacco and lung cancer also published in 1950 resembled that of the two American case–control studies I characterized as naive in the previous section. The study was conducted in 1948 and 1949. The study's group of cases consisted of 649 male patients admitted for lung cancer in twenty London hospitals. A control who was free of lung cancer but of the same sex, age, and hospital location was selected for each lung cancer case. Both case and control groups were asked identical questions regarding how long they had been smoking, dates of starting and stopping cigarette and pipe smoking, and the amount smoked. Why was this study better designed, though?

Before I address this question, let's linger on another interesting aspect of the report: the definition of a smoker. By the time of the study, tobacco smoking had become so prevalent that a preliminary step was to define who was a smoker. How would you define a smoker? Would you include, for example, a woman who had one cigarette annually after her Christmas dinner? Or a fifty-year-old man who as a youth had smoked a couple of cigarettes to see if he liked it and decided he did not? Positive answers to these two questions yield an overly inclusive definition, which in 1950 would have described everyone as a smoker. There had to be an exposure threshold distinguishing smokers from nonsmokers.

Doll and Hill defined an "ever smoker" as a person who had smoked as much as one cigarette a day for as long as one year or, for pipe smokers, at least seven grams of tobacco per week for as long as a year. Any less consistent amount was ignored. According to this definition, have you ever been a smoker? The smoking histories obtained were, of course, a function of the patient's memory and veracity. To test their recall accuracy, fifty people were asked the same question twice, six months apart: "How much did you smoke before the onset of your present illness?" They provided almost identical answers both times. This was reassuring.

In the Doll and Hill study, 647 of the 649 lung cancer cases (that is, 99.7 percent) and 622 of the 649 controls (that is, 95.8 percent) had smoked. Not a terribly impressive difference to say the least. In both groups, the vast majority of men had smoked. Only 2 (0.3 percent) of the cases versus 27 (4.2 percent) of the controls had never smoked![18] I am sure you would not be convinced that this was a meaningful difference, but who would be?

This is precisely where Doll and Hill had an ingenious idea. They knew that just before being admitted into a hospital, their cases and controls were some of the 4 million men who lived in London at that time, pursuing their usual life and indulging in their smoking habits. Then they assumed that over about eighteen months all those Londoners who developed lung cancer would have been hospitalized and therefore recruited into their study. Thus, had they known the smoking habits of each of the 4 million male Londoners, they could have compared the risk of lung cancer of the smokers and the nonsmokers. They would have divided the number of lung cancer cases in their study by the number of Londoners, separately for the smokers and the nonsmokers. That would have been ideal, but obtaining the smoking habits of 4 million men in 1950 was science fiction. Thus, Doll and Hill made a second bold assumption: if the diseases among the controls were not caused by tobacco, their smoking habits had to be similar to those of the 4 million Londoners, and therefore their 649 controls were equivalent to a representative sample of the same 4 million Londoners from whom the cases came. We know today that this second assumption was unwarranted. Tobacco smoking is more prevalent in hospitalized populations than in their community of origin because it is harmful in many different ways. But the assumption allowed Doll and Hill to estimate the number of smokers among a much larger group of 4 million men.

They deduced that because 95.8 percent of the controls smoked, it was likely that the same percentage, 95.8, of male Londoners smoked as well: so 95.8 percent of 4 million is 3,832,000 men. Thus, the risk of developing lung cancer among smokers can be estimated by dividing 647 lung cancer cases of smokers by 3,832,000 smokers. This makes 0.00017 or 17 per 100,000 smokers. And for the nonsmokers, the risk is estimated by dividing the 2 cases of lung cancer in the nonsmokers by 168,000 (4.2 percent of the 4 million male Londoners), which is 1.2 per 100,000.

Now, the ratio of these two risks (17 ÷ 1.2) was 14.2, meaning that smokers had fourteen times more risk than nonsmokers for developing lung cancer. This risk ratio was even greater for heavy smokers and for moderate smokers compared to never smokers. Does this convince you that there is an association? Doll and Hill firmly concluded that smoking is "a factor, and an important factor, in the production of carcinoma of the lung."[19]

Admittedly, going from a small difference in the proportion of smokers among cases and among controls (99.7 percent and 95.8 percent) to a ratio of 14.2 using the same data looks like the result of a magic trick. And, indeed, it may have left many perplexed in the 1950s. It is therefore not surprising that even this clever way of conducting case–control studies did not suffice in the quest to demonstrate the causative role of tobacco in lung cancer.

## PROFESSOR CORNFIELD AND REVEREND BAYES

There was a key assumption in the way Doll and Hill had computed their risk ratios: the ability to claim that the control group's smoking habits were

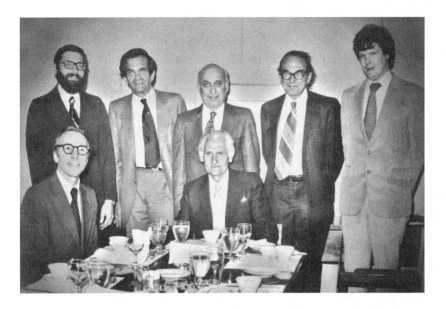

FIGURE 7.2

Participants to an epidemiology symposium in 1979. The photograph was taken at the offices of the American Health Foundation in the building of the Ford Foundation, New York, 1979. *Sitting, left to right:* Arthur Upton and Sir Richard Doll. *Standing, left to right:* Steven D. Stellman, Ernst L. Wynder, Lester Breslow, Jerome Cornfield, and Harland Austin. (Courtesy of Steven D. Stellman)

similar to those of Greater London inhabitants. It is rare that case–control studies meet this assumption, however. Neither Wynder and Graham nor Levin and his collaborators could have related their control group to a larger, well-defined, and enumerated population.

Jerome Cornfield successively served as president of the American Epidemiologic Society and the American Statistical Association (figure 7.2). He therefore had the respect of both epidemiologists and statisticians. In 1951, he showed mathematically that there was a connection between the history of smoking in cases and controls and the risk of lung cancer in smokers and nonsmokers. As mentioned earlier, if people who developed lung cancer had smoked more in the past than comparable people who had remained free of lung cancer, it was logical to expect that it was for this reason that they had been more likely to develop lung cancer.[20] For this demonstration, Cornfield used an old but still widely used theorem attributed to the English reverend Thomas Bayes in the mid–eighteenth century. Applying the theorem in the context of a group comparison, he demonstrated that there was a way of combining the two proportions of smokers (among the cases and the controls) that would yield a close approximation of the risk ratio of lung cancer. Appendix 2 provides a technical explanation.

Let us apply Cornfield's idea to the results of Doll and Hill's study. The frequencies of ever smokers were 99.7 and 95.8 percent, and the frequencies of never smokers were 0.3 and 4.2 percent. These percentages can be transformed into an odds ratio of 14.6 (99.7/0.3 ÷ 95.8/4.2). (See appendix 2.) The odds ratio of 14.6 is slightly larger than the risk ratio of 14.2. Some of the differences come from imprecision in the computations. The key point is that the odds ratio and the risk ratio can be interpreted in the same way: smokers are about fourteen times more at risk of developing lung cancer than nonsmokers.

Thus, thanks to Cornfield's new approach, the results of a case–control study can be interpreted in terms of a risk ratio. In Doll and Hill's study, 99.7 percent of the lung cancer cases and 95.8 percent of the controls were smokers, which corresponded to a risk of lung cancer in smokers fourteen times greater than the risk for nonsmokers!

## THE BRITISH DOCTORS STUDY

By 1951, a number of new case–control studies, in addition to those described in this chapter, had been performed on the smoking habits of patients with and without lung cancer. Further studies of the same kind were unlikely to convince the persistent skeptics that the association between smoking and lung cancer was causal. Nevertheless, the sufficient amount of evidence showing a possible association between cigarettes and lung cancer generated by the various case–control studies justified the need for much larger studies to directly observe whether smokers were at higher risk of lung cancer than nonsmokers.

Bradford Hill proposed to query a large number of individuals about their smoking habits, follow them forward in time, and determine whether the cigarette smokers among them would have a higher mortality from lung cancer than the nonsmokers.

[Exposed cohort] Smokers ⟶ follow up ⟶ lung cancer

[Nonexposed cohort] Nonsmokers ⟶ follow up ⟶ lung cancer

Lung cancer was by the 1950s much more common than it was at the beginning of the twentieth century, but even with rates as high as 40 per 100,000 per year it remained a relatively rare disease. In, say, ten years of follow-up, 200 new cases would occur from 50,000 people whose smoking habits would be known. In addition, following such a large group of people for multiple years raised technical and logistical problems. In the 1950s, all research had to be done using paper-and-pencil questionnaires, mail correspondence, and Hollerith punch cards. Still no computer.

Bradford Hill devised an ideal study population: doctors. There were approximately 60,000 doctors in the United Kingdom who belonged to the British Medical Association, were educated, and could be motivated. The British Medical Register offered a convenient way of tracking each doctor's current location and vital status across time. These conditions were optimal for following a large number of people over a long period of time, enumerating deaths and their causes, and, it was hoped, losing a minimal number of study subjects over time.

In October 1951, the 59,600 men and women on the current British Medical Register and residing in the United Kingdom received a short and simple questionnaire. Besides name, address, and age, it asked the doctors if they still smoked tobacco, if they had previously smoked but had given it up, or if they had never regularly smoked cigarettes, pipes, or cigars. The current and former smokers were also asked to indicate amounts smoked and chronology. The totality of the questionnaire is reproduced here. I invite you to answer it for yourself.

Are you a smoker?

Note.—For the purpose of this inquiry a person is deemed to be a smoker if he has ever smoked as much as one cigarette per day for as long as one year

Section 1: PRESENT SMOKERS

(a) I began smoking regularly when aged _____

(b) At the present time my consumption of tobacco is about

_____ cigarettes a day
_____ ounces of tobacco a week in home-made cigarettes
_____ ounces of tobacco a week in a pipe

(c) My age last birthday was _____

OR

Section 2: EX-SMOKERS

(a) I began smoking regularly when aged _____

When I last gave up I was aged _____

(b) My consumption of tobacco at the time I last gave up smoking was about:
_____ cigarettes a day
_____ ounces of tobacco a week in home-made cigarettes
_____ ounces of tobacco a week in a pipe

(c) My age last birthday was _____

OR

Section 3: NON-SMOKERS

(a) Please tick the appropriate statement

I have never smoked at all
I have had an occasional smoke

(b) My age last birthday was _____ [21]

Two out of three British doctors in 1951 filled out the first section, whereas you most likely completed sections 2 or 3. Times have changed.

About 40,000 doctors replied: 34,000 men and 6,000 women. In other words, 69 percent of the male and 60 percent of the female living doctors in the United Kingdom participated in the inquiry.[22] They were allocated to nonsmoking or smoking categories according to their initial replies in 1951 and followed thereafter. Of course, many doctors changed smoking habits after 1951 and, in particular, stopped smoking. How would you classify them? You may consider adapting their smoking status all along the way. But some of the changes in smoking habits may have been the consequence of the doctors becoming sick from their smoking habits. In that case, the smoking habit is the consequence of disease, whereas the study is designed to assess whether disease is the consequence of the smoking habit. It is terribly important in cohort studies to clearly separate the period when exposure is assessed from the period when cases of disease are identified.

The British Doctors Study assessed the impact of tobacco consumption on deaths from lung cancer. Each time the British Medical Association recorded having lost one of the study participants, the death certificate was obtained. This method ensured that all of the deaths were identified and did not go unnoticed.

This group comparison compared doctors who had ever regularly smoked at least one cigarette per day before 1951 with doctors who had not. Recall that today we call this design a "cohort study," but then it was called a "prospective" study because it began by measuring the incriminated cause (smoking) and went forward in time to assess the associated risk of disease.

Why, might you ask, am I calling this "cohort" study conducted among British doctors "new," considering that we saw in chapter 6 that Wilhelm Weinberg had conducted one in Germany half a century earlier? I do so because the British doctors filled out a questionnaire in person and were followed during their lifetime, whereas Weinberg worked with information stored in registries and had no contact with his study participants.

After ten years of follow-up, there were (only) 212 deaths from lung cancer in men and 6 in women. Figure 7.3 shows the contrast between ever and never smokers of cigarettes. Lung cancer was rare among doctors who had never smoked cigarettes.

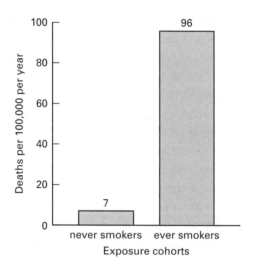

FIGURE 7.3 **Annual Risk of Dying from Lung Cancer, 1951–1961**

British Doctors Study comparing the mortality rates from lung cancer (per 100,000 doctors and per year). Exposure to tobacco was determined in 1951: 5,439 doctors had never
smoked, and 18,060 were current or former cigarette smokers ("ever smokers"). After
ten years of follow-up, there were among the never smokers 3 cases of lung cancer for
42,860 person-years and among the ever smokers 143 cases of lung cancer for 149,000
person-years.                                                          *Source*: Doll and Hill 1964.

## SMOKERS' TRUE RISK

Not all the doctors were followed for ten full years. A doctor who died
in 1952, for example, had been in the study for only one year, whereas a
doctor still alive in 1961 had been in the study for ten years. There was a
need for a way to take into account only the duration of follow-up during
which each participant was materially at risk of developing lung cancer.
Doll and Hill's solution was to compute the total number of years the
40,000 doctors had been in the study, transforming persons into person-
years.[23] One person followed for two years represented two person-years,
like two persons followed for one year each. Doll and Hill then divided
the number of lung cancer cases by person-years and obtained mortality

rates from lung cancer per year. Lung cancer was rare among nonsmokers: 7 cases were diagnosed for each 100,000 people followed for one year. The mortality rate was about 100 per 100,000 per year among smokers.

On the basis of these two rates, how can we quantify the harm? Both rates are expressed in the same way, per 100,000 persons per year. The ratio is therefore $100 \div 7 = 14.3$, or 14! Ever smokers are fourteen times more likely than never smokers to die from lung cancer. Does this number ring a bell? It is also the value of the risk ratio computed by Doll and Hill in their "ingenious" case–control study.

Are you not impressed that two study designs apparently so different—the comparison of cases of lung cancer with controls free of lung cancer and the follow-up of smokers and nonsmokers over ten years—led to almost exactly the same risk ratio of 14? Actually, this identity of ratios is expected because the cohort and the case–control studies use different approaches to address the same question. Conceptually, the cohort study represents a cause-to-effect approach, tracking the occurrence of lung cancer among smokers and nonsmokers, whereas the case–control study is an effect-to-cause approach that consists in determining the past smoking habits of people who developed lung cancer and those who did not. Appendix 3 provides a more formal explanation for why cohort and case–control studies concur.

Note that a mortality rate of 1 per 1,000 per year is not telling for a smoker. It sounds small, and it is hard to visualize what it means over a lifetime. An individual would rather like to know what the risk of dying from lung cancer is if one keeps smoking for many years. How would you rework the mortality rates measured in the British Doctors Study into long-term risks that are meaningful for the individual? A simple way to approximate these risks is to assume that the average rate applies over a long period of time. For example, the forty-five-year risk among ever smokers is about 4.5 percent ($45 \times 0.001$). What is the forty-five-year risk for a never smoker?[24] What is the forty-five-year risk for a smoker of a pack or more per day given that the average mortality rate in the British Doctors Study was 227 per 100,000 per year? It is 10 percent! Hence, the popular notion that a never smoker has a low risk of developing lung cancer, whereas a smoker of a pack or more per day has a 10 percent risk of developing lung cancer over his or her lifetime.

## SMOKERS' LONGEVITY

The British Doctors Study has been a sustained source of knowledge on the health effects of tobacco use. The doctors were easily traced. After twenty years, only 103 out of the original 34,440 men (0.3 percent) were unaccounted for. Analyses were published every ten years. The 2004 publication reported results after fifty years of follow-up, from 1951 to 2001.[25] Concerns moved from the mortality from lung cancer, which did not have to be demonstrated anymore, to the general survival of smokers.

How long do smokers and never smokers live?

This is an impressive result of the British Doctors Study: half of the heavy cigarette smokers (of twenty-five or more cigarettes a day) died before age seventy compared to 20 percent of never smokers. Less than one out of every ten heavy smokers survived to the age of eighty-five compared to one out of every three never smokers. In average, heavy smoking took away ten years of life, sometimes by cancer, but mostly by heart and chronic respiratory diseases.

The results of the British Doctors Study have been confirmed by subsequent research. Mortality from lung cancer increases with the number of cigarettes smoked daily. There is no threshold under which tobacco smoking is safe. One cigarette a day impacts lung cancer risk. Among heavy smokers, the relation to lung cancer is so strong that it cannot be explained by any other cause than the content of tobacco smoke. Equally striking and informative is that mortality rapidly decreases after smoking cessation. Twenty years after smoking cessation, former and never smokers have the same very low risk of lung cancer.

The British Doctors Study is a fabulously successful piece of research, whose results are consistent with most of the current health knowledge on the long-term risks of consuming tobacco and long-term benefits of smoking cessation.

## CONTROVERSY

In 1950, some scientists were unconvinced by the results of group comparisons indicating a link between tobacco and lung cancer. Among these critics was the statistician Ronald A. Fisher in Cambridge in the United Kingdom.[26]

## The Smoking Gene

Fisher first criticized Doll and Hill for failing to take into consideration what he believed was the true cause of the relation of tobacco to lung cancer: a smoking gene. Fisher argued that smokers were genetically attracted to tobacco.

To support his thesis, he presented data about the smoking habits of identical and fraternal twins. Monozygotic twins (twins whose genetic constitution is almost identical because they come from a single egg that splits into two) were more alike in their smoking behavior than dizygotic twins (fraternal twins who have only half of their genes in common because they come from two separate eggs). Among fifty-one identical twin pairs, 76 percent had similar smoking habits, as opposed to 48 percent of the thirty-one fraternal twin pairs. For Fisher, that meant that genes influenced whether you smoked or not.

The second component of Fisher's argument was that cancer itself was a genetic disease. Therefore, the relation between smoking and lung cancer that Doll and Hill had observed was in fact an indirect link. Instead, Fisher claimed that the real culprit was none other than a genetic component not assessed by Doll and Hill.

Doll and Hill observed the following association:

smoking ⟶ lung cancer

Fisher believed that smoking and lung cancer appeared to be related in case–control studies because they had a common genetic cause.

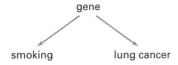

According to Fisher's theory, Doll and Hill mistook cigarettes for the cause of lung cancer because they neglected the genetic factor.

Doll and Hill refuted Fisher's argument. A genetic cause could not explain the 22 percent growth of the mortality from lung cancer among English men age twenty-five and older between 1952 and 1962. It also could not explain why, during the same period, mortality from cancer of the lung among the doctors of the British Doctors Study had fallen. Which smoking gene could increase smoking prevalence and mortality in the population and decrease it among doctors?

## When Inhaling Protects

Fisher also delved into an incoherent aspect of the case–control study by Doll and Hill: 62 percent of the lung cancer cases versus 67 percent of the controls free of lung cancer reported inhaling tobacco smoke. Following the logic of the case–control comparison, if inhalation of tobacco were more common among those who did not develop lung cancer than among those who did, it could mean inhaling was potentially protective against lung cancer.

Doll and Hill were stunned by this paradoxical result. Was it a consequence of chronic bronchitis and emphysema among smokers that their ability to inhale was hampered? Fisher sarcastically jibed that this implied that 10 percent of lung cancer cases could be prevented if smokers inhaled more often: "[I]nhalers may congratulate themselves on reducing the cancer incidence by over 10 percent, using a very simple, and even enjoyable method of prevention."[27]

Back-up support for Doll and Hill, however, came from a French study published in 1961.[28] This study confirmed the relation of tobacco smoke to lung cancer with cases of lung cancer reporting more inhalation than the controls.[29]

## THE SCIENTIFIC AND SOCIAL IMPACT

By the mid-1960s, after more than ten years of controversy, an official position on the question regarding the health effects of tobacco use was badly needed: Is cigarette smoking a cause of lung cancer? In 1962, an English Royal College of Physicians report entitled *Smoking and Health* answered affirmatively. The Americans followed in 1964, but the way they reached their conclusion is a milestone in the history of public health.

## The Causality Viewpoints

US surgeon general Luther Terry was in charge of settling the issue. In 1963, the positions of the tobacco industry and of the scientists who had accrued the evidence about the health damages of tobacco seemed irreconcilable. Huge economic interests were at stake. Legal claims from smokers against the cigarette manufacturers had so far failed but were still a threat to the industry's profitability. Nonetheless, Terry assembled an advisory committee that could be granted tobacco industry approval.[30] Not only did two of the committee members represent the various cigarette manufacturers, but they also had their say in the selection of the other members. Among the independent scientists, there was a single epidemiologist, a heavy smoker from the University of Minnesota, Leonard M. Schuman, who had not been directly involved in previous publications on the health effects of tobacco.[31]

Regardless of the committee's makeup, its members faced a tough challenge. The question of whether tobacco caused cancer had no simple solution. How would you have proceeded had you received Terry's mandate? Tobacco was not strychnine. Smokers do not fall dead within hours. In fact, only a small minority of those who smoke get cancer.

The committee met for thirteen months to examine the evidence. It noted that the risk of dying from cancer of the lung in heavy cigarette smokers was twenty to thirty times greater than that of never smokers; that lung cancer was rare among never smokers; that the more someone smoked, the higher the risk of lung cancer; that studies conducted in many different populations of the world consistently found the same deleterious effects of smoking. For example, of the twenty-nine case–control studies, all but one conducted among women confirmed the association. All these different viewpoints incriminated tobacco use as the culprit. They convinced the committee members.

Finally, in 1964, Surgeon General Terry announced the unanimous conclusion of his consulting committee: "Cigarette smoking is causally related to lung cancer in men."[32] This report represented a historical milestone of greater significance than any previous document on the topic had ever achieved. It established the connection between tobacco and disease in the public's eye and offered a body of medical evidence that could be used in court to support claims of harm. Any rebuttal constrained the defendants to argue against the US surgeon general.

## The Alliance of Epidemiology and Law

The immediate public-health consequences of the surgeon general's report were limited. Cigarette sales plunged briefly after 1964 but soon recuperated.

However, the knowledge about the adverse health effects of smoking fueled nonsmokers' suspicions. In rooms filled with smoke, did nonsmokers breathe cancer-causing tobacco constituents? Did passive smoking also increase risk? Some studies showed an increase of 30 percent (risk ratio = 1.3).

The threat of passive smoking had a tremendous public-health impact, much larger than what followed from the revelations of the surgeon general's report.

The tobacco industry had easily attenuated the congressional regulatory activity that followed the 1964 surgeon general's report by claiming that smoking was an adult choice and adults were free to do what they wanted. This logic failed, however, when it was argued that smokers imperiled the health of their nonsmoking wives, children, and people in their surroundings. There was matter for litigation.

An epic campaign against the tobacco corporations led by a heterogeneous coalition of antitobacco activists, lawyers, politicians, and state attorneys general began. A famous and successful trial started in 1992. It led to the recognition that tobacco smoke had innocent victims.

Flight attendants who served in smoke-filled cabins of airplanes for years developed lung cancer even though they were nonsmokers. In 1991, they filed a class action against Philip Morris. The named tobacco companies agreed to pay $300 million to establish an institute supporting research on tobacco smoke and health.

Additional class-action suits filed against tobacco companies evolved into coordinated action by several states. They always ended up in agreements in which the industry agreed to pay hundreds of millions of dollars to settle in order to avoid what it feared the most: an antitobacco law. In 1998, US states and territories signed the Master Settlement Agreement with the four largest tobacco companies, which agreed to pay $200 billion over a twenty-five-year period.

The history of the mass litigation against the tobacco industry in the United States is fascinating because it shows that American attorneys did not take long to understand the role of epidemiology. Trials are won with evidence. For health matters, this evidence stems from group comparisons. The industry could pretend that tobacco is harmless for health. The presiding judge might be a smoker himself, with many friends who smoked and lived to an advanced age, and might not believe that tobacco caused cancer. But here was the evidence: the comparison of thousands of smokers and nonsmokers indicated that tobacco increased the risk of cancer.

Trials were won by the complainants, and tobacco smoking was progressively banned from workplaces, public places, bars, and restaurants, then later in residential buildings and public parks in the United States, and then elsewhere.[33]

## WORK IN PROGRESS

The history of the cigarette has been brilliantly written by others.[34] I won't summarize it here. Let's simply consider the riveting, almost symmetrical evolution of US cigarette sales between 1900 and 2005, as shown in figure 7.8. The number of cigarettes sold per American in 2005 was similar to that of 1935. Between these two dates, a formidable rise and decline of the smoking epidemic occurred. The apex was reached in 1965. Something clearly happened in the 1950s and 1960s to invert the historical trend in cigarette consumption. Death rates from lung cancer began to decline between 1990 and 2000 among men and sometime between 2003 and 2007 among women.[35]

Although tobacco use in Western societies is no longer what it used to be in the 1950s and 1960s, the prevention of tobacco smoking remains an important issue on the agenda, especially in low-income and middle-income countries. In 2010, half of the men and one in every ten women

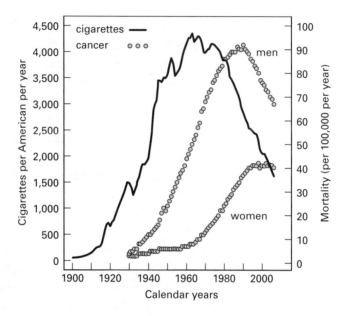

FIGURE 7.4 **Cigarettes per Person (1900–2006) and
Deaths from Lung Cancer (1930–2006) in the United States**

Evolution of the number of cigarettes sold and mortality from lung cancer in the United
States between 1900 and 2006. The figure also indicates that prevention of tobacco smoking remains on the agenda. In 2006, 1,619 cigarettes per person per year were still sold
in the United States.

*Source*: Compiled from data given at various Centers for Disease Control
and Prevention and US Department of Agriculture websites.

still used tobacco in Bangladesh, Brazil, China, Egypt, India, Mexico, Phil-
ippines, Poland, Russia, Thailand, Turkey, Ukraine, Uruguay, and Viet-
nam,[36] representing about a billion tobacco users.

Yet the use of epidemiology by scientists and lawyers in the United
States dismantled the unjustifiable illusions about the health benefits
of cigarettes that characterized the first half of the twentieth century.
The label on cigarette packs, "Smoking Kills," is the legal translation of
the epidemiologic observation that smokers die earlier than nonsmokers. The warning label "Smoking causes heart disease, lung cancer, and

emphysema" is the legal translation of the epidemiologic observation that the risk of heart disease, lung cancer, and emphysema is greater among smokers than among nonsmokers. These are matters of evidence based on data from group comparisons, case–control studies, and cohort studies, which were refined to meet the challenge of studying the effects of tobacco on health.

The controversy and the battle regarding the effects of tobacco use on health has been the great worksite of epidemiology. Epidemiology thereafter emerged as a preeminent scientific discipline, with its own theories, journals, university departments, and textbooks.[37]

Before you finish this chapter, you may want to know what happened to the other main hypothesis about lung cancer. Were engine exhaust and fumes from road tar exonerated from all responsibility in cancer causation? Nope. Work on the relationship between air pollution from engine exhaust and lung cancer is still in progress. You may have read, for example, the many news reports in June 2012 that announced in their headlines, "Diesel Engine Exhaust Causes Lung Cancer, WHO Agency Says." The conclusion was based on group comparisons conducted in particular among workers.

# 8

# DAILY LIFE MYSTERIES
# AND EPIDEMIOLOGY

SINCE 1965, the contribution of epidemiology has soared. The proliferation of group comparisons in medicine and public health precludes tracking the historical evolution of epidemiology from a few milestone studies as in earlier days. However, most of the group comparisons appear to have been used to answer five types of scientific questions: Is this treatment dangerous? Is this treatment effective? What is the optimal medical decision? Is there a health risk or a health benefit? Is this screening effective? These questions are very much part of our daily life. They lack the historical luster of the enigmas about the plague, the blue death, tuberculosis, and lung cancer. Nevertheless, they are the modern scientific mysteries that epidemiology contributes to unraveling.

Here briefly and in chapters 9 through 13 more thoroughly, I deal with these questions approximately in the chronological order of their emergence (there is of course much overlap) and illustrate them with significant studies—also organized as much as possible chronologically.

## IS THIS TREATMENT DANGEROUS
## FOR HEALTH?

The ability of epidemiology to evaluate the dangerousness of treatment proved useful when, after the Second World War, medical practice rapidly incorporated technological innovations in diagnostic tests and treatments.

Before 1950, doctors had few effective drugs. After 1950, many new drugs appeared on the market, some of which had, obviously, considerable adverse effects. A course of streptomycin, for example, the first effective treatment for tuberculosis, could be terribly painful. The British novelist George Orwell gave in his last notebook a lucid and poignant description of how adverse effects forced him to prematurely interrupt his treatment.[1]

Orwell's suffering was not isolated. Numerous novel diagnostic tests and surgical and medical treatments were dangerous for health. They surprised Robert Moser when, as chief of the Department of Medicine in a small US Army hospital in Austria, he was presented with three patients in a row who suffered from symptoms that seemed caused by the drugs they were taking. Moser began a collection of scientific evidence about adverse effects of therapies and in September 1956 summarized his findings in the *New England Journal of Medicine*.[2] The article soon became a book, *Diseases of Medical Progress*,[3] whose third edition, in 1969, distilled eight hundred pages of "iatrogenic diseases," a term that come from the Greek *iatros*, which means "doctor"—that is, diseases caused by the medical prescription of drugs, surgery, or diagnostic procedures.[4]

Streptomycin was effective, but other new treatments were not even that. Alvan Feinstein, an American pioneer of group comparisons in medicine, which he called "clinical epidemiology," noted in his 1967 book *Clinical Judgment* that numerous medical errors had resulted from an uncritical integration of treatments. He mentioned removal of the uterus to cure nonspecific backaches; surgical attachment of the stomach or kidney to the abdominal wall or to the diaphragm to treat the descent of these organs from their normal positions; total extraction of teeth for rheumatoid fever; mismatched blood transfusions; radiotherapy for acne, which resulted in skin cancer; and thalidomide treatment of morning sickness in pregnant women, which caused developmental anomalies in their fetuses. All of these unfortunate therapeutic procedures, Feinstein stressed, had been carried out by "well-intentioned, honest, dedicated, apparently enlightened clinicians working with the scientific diagnostic methods and therapeutic agents of modern medicine."[5]

What was wrong? Clinical medicine was lacking a method to assess the efficacy of the new procedures and identify their potential complications.

A mysterious doctor-made epidemic was going on, and epidemiology was used to successfully solve some of its most tragic enigmas.

Chapter 9 delves into two, highly publicized examples. In the international scandal of the drug thalidomide, the crippling effects of the drug were so spectacular that they were identified with a form of comparison that we have not previously discussed, consisting of comparing the observed frequency of congenital malformation with the frequency that would have been expected in the same population (1961). In the second example, about the death of young women in whom a Dalkon Shield intrauterine device had been implanted for contraceptive purpose, a case–control study nabbed the device as being responsible (1983).

## DOES THE TREATMENT WORK?

Doctors have long been skeptical about the use of group comparisons in clinical medicine. They rightly believed that no two patients were alike. Grouping patients to focus on what they had in common implied ignoring what made each patient special. Group comparisons, therefore, could not capture the richness and complexity that doctors could perceive when they examined the patient.

Nevertheless, an indubitable convergence of epidemiology and clinical medicine occurred during the last decades of the twentieth century. The invention of randomized controlled trials (RCTs) played a decisive role in converting doctors to epidemiology.

### The Randomized Controlled Trial

In its most simple form, the RCT consists of allocating an experimental treatment and a control treatment to study subjects by a chance-based procedure equivalent to the toss of a coin. For instance, say that one hundred people have agreed to participate in a trial. A coin is tossed for each of them. If it lands heads up, the person gets the experimental treatment. If it comes up tails, the person gets the control treatment. Thanks to this allocation procedure, about fifty people will be randomly assigned the experimental treatment. More importantly, *on average*, the characteristics of these people, such as their mean age, sex, mean weight, and so on will tend to be identical or very similar to the other fifty people who will receive the control treatment.

Thus, properly performed for a sufficiently large number of patients, the process of randomly allocating treatments produces groups that are exchangeable in every aspect, such as age, gender, ethnicity, and so on. The only difference is that one of the groups receives the experimental treatment that the study intends to assess.

Why call it a "randomized controlled trial"? The term *trial* means "experiment." Trials are usually performed in laboratories, but in this case it is a human experiment that does not necessarily take place in a laboratory. The qualifier *controlled* stresses the fact that it is a group comparison with one group serving as the control. The modifier *randomized* refers to the chance procedure, such as the fair toss of a coin, used to allocate the treatment.

The invention of the RCT has given medicine a technique to perform group comparisons, which, more than with any other methods, guarantees the comparability of the groups: well-conducted randomization makes comparable groups.

## Cochrane Collaboration

RCTs may not have been adopted so rapidly by doctors had young physicians not seen in it a way of improving health justice. Archibald Cochrane was instrumental in this respect. In 1972, he proposed to use RCTs systematically to distinguish treatments and medical procedures that worked from those that did not. If the UK National Health Service, he explained, did not have to pay for ineffective treatments, it could use the savings to ensure a greater equity towards effective treatments. Therapeutic efficacy would therefore go hand in hand with social justice.[6] The 1970s were years in which universities, including medical schools, were preoccupied with ideas of social progress. Cochrane's vision of using epidemiology to attenuate the social inequalities in access to health care rallied many young epidemiologists to this cause.

In 1979, Cochrane further observed: "It is surely a great criticism of our profession that we have not organized a critical summary, by specialty or subspecialty, adapted periodically, of all relevant randomized controlled trials."[7] To separate good care from chaff, a critical synthesis of all RCTs testing the effectiveness of a treatment would generate a global message that carried a weight greater than the results of individual studies.

Under the leadership of Sir Iain Chalmers, an obstetrician and health services researcher in Oxford, the 1987 Oxford Database of Perinatal Trials was developed, the result of an international collaboration and "a real milestone in the history of randomized trials and in the evaluation of care" according to Cochrane.[8] The extension of this collaborative model in perinatal epidemiology to other medical domains led to the establishment of the Cochrane Collaboration in 1993.

Thousands of Cochrane reviews are now available to medical practitioners and the general public. The Cochrane Collaboration website, www.cochrane.org, has made its contents easily accessible. The Cochrane Library already includes more than 4,000 reviews about the efficacy of therapeutic and preventive interventions. One can find analyses of topics as diverse as drugs, vitamins, acupuncture, St. John's wort, and vaccines. Each has a technical summary and a summary for the general public, followed by the results of studies shown in a standardized format. Sometimes an audio track of the author explains in lay terms the review's aims, its results, and its conclusions.

I often start with Cochrane reviews when I am looking for an answer to a question about a treatment or about a means of prevention.[9] On its home page, the Cochrane Collaboration proudly quotes a statement by *The Lancet*: "The Cochrane Collaboration is an enterprise that rivals the Human Genome Project in its potential implications for modern medicine." The Cochrane Collaboration claims 28,000 participants conducting reviews in 110 countries.[10]

Chapter 10 begins by reviewing the technical mistakes that plagued the early RCTs until researchers finally learned how to conduct them well (1898–1938). The famous streptomycin trial (1948) was probably the first of these well-conducted trials to have a large echo in the medical community. The group receiving streptomycin was compared with another group only confined to bed rest. The trial offers, therefore, an opportunity to discuss the discovery of the placebo effect, which became a systematic concern later on. Chapter 10 also revisits a classic controversy that surrounded one of the first evaluations of a drug to treat the acquired immune deficiency syndrome (AIDS), azidothymidine (AZT), in the Concord trial (1994). The discord over Concorde engendered a controversy about the interpretation of RCTs performed under suboptimal technical conditions and, in particular, when the composition of the randomized groups had been severely compromised.

## WHAT IS THE OPTIMAL MEDICAL DECISION?

Using epidemiology, in particular the findings of group comparisons, to single out the optimal medical decision for a patient took place in medicine during the last quarter of the twentieth century. The idea was to borrow what had been learned in population studies to inform the decisions regarding individual patients. The mass of epidemiologic information was already large in the 1970s. It has become mind-boggling today. Techniques were therefore invented to help doctors access and organize this information in a meaningful way.

### Clinical Decision Analysis

In the 1970s, a small group of clinicians invented "clinical decision analysis," also known as "medical decision analysis."[11] Their basic idea was to use epidemiologic data from the medical literature to sort out which of several possible therapeutic decisions was potentially associated with the greatest benefit for an individual patient. Clinical decision analysis was deemed particularly useful for the situations in which the clinical management of individual patients did not seem to suffice. These were situations in which doctors often erred. Appendicitis was a typical example. In the presence of pain in the right lower abdomen, clinicians were often ambivalent as to whether they should immediately prescribe surgery to remove an inflamed appendix (and impose an unwarranted surgical procedure) or wait some hours to see whether the patient improved without surgery (and take the risk of a serious, life-threatening complication of appendicitis). Suspicion of pulmonary embolism was another of these clinical situations in which clinicians felt that they could flip a coin to choose among several decisions.

In hindsight, clinical decision analysis had only a marginal impact on clinical practice.[12] It lacks flexibility. It can take days to weeks to generate a qualified strategy. The fate of the patient might have long been sealed. Nevertheless, in its attempt to reconcile clinical judgment, the results of RCTs, and other quantitative data from the medical literature in an explicit and understandable clinical strategy, it has contributed to familiarizing clinicians with epidemiology and has paved the way for "evidence-based medicine" (EBM).

Chapter 11 builds on the case of a hypothetical doctor struggling with the management of patients whom she suspects suffered from pulmonary embolism to illustrate how clinical decision analysis can help clinicians identify the optimal medical decision for each individual patient. Pulmonary embolism typified these stealthy clinical syndromes for which modern doctors suddenly had access to a variety of diagnostic and therapeutic options (1976).

## Evidence-Based Medicine

EBM has just emerged from its teenage years. In 1993, the *Journal of the American Medical Association*—better known by its acronym *JAMA*—published a series of papers from the working group on EBM.[13] The group envisioned a medical practice that combined "conscientiously, explicitly, judiciously" numerical data gathered from populations of patients and clinical expertise accrued in the management of individual patients. EBM required that physicians learn how to integrate results derived from group comparisons into their clinical judgments and decisions.[14]

Thanks to EBM, clinicians gained access to epidemiology in an unprecedented way. Before 1980, epidemiologic methods and concepts, with the exception of the theory of RCTs, focused mainly on public-health issues. The textbooks, the terminology, and the examples belonged to public health and did not interest medical students or doctors. Clinical epidemiology—that is, the application of epidemiology to clinical practice—existed, but its supporters were few. EBM reformulated the concepts and changed the terminology and examples in order to adapt epidemiology to medical practice. It gave clinical epidemiology an unprecedented impetus.

Before the advent of pocket computers, the EBM manual, sized as a breviary that can be carried in the hospital doctor's white coat, was an epidemiologically driven treatise on how to synthesize medical evidence.

Since EBM is also a way of analyzing and interpreting the results of group comparisons, Chapter 11 invites you to apply EBM tools to the results of an RCT concerning the efficacy of a vaginal gel in preventing HIV infection (2010).

## HEALTH RISK OR BENEFIT?

The elucidation of the causal role of tobacco for lung cancer is the classic example of the contribution of epidemiology to establishing health risk (see chapter 7). To build a cogent argument, epidemiologists refined the methodology of case–control and cohort studies and better understood the theory that connects these two study designs.

Since 1950, epidemiology has identified a wealth of other health risks. In 2005, Diana Petitti listed some of these associations.[15] It was found that tobacco alone increased the risk of lung cancer, heart attacks, stroke, cancer of the larynx and esophagus (especially when combined with alcohol), and slow fetal growth; Hepatitis B virus caused liver cancer; Epstein-Barr virus caused Burkitt and nasopharyngeal cancer; a herpes virus (type 8) caused Kaposi's sarcoma; human papilloma virus caused cervical cancer; tampons caused toxic shock syndrome (before the causal staphylococcus bacterium was identified); asbestos and uranium radon caused lung cancer; aniline dye caused bladder cancer (in particular among smokers); gaseous nickel caused respiratory cancers; and vinyl chloride caused angiosarcoma of the liver. Group comparisons also showed the familial aggregation of breast, ovarian, and colon cancers before the discovery of the genes BRCA1, BRCA2, and APC1.

Another novelty was the adaptation of the principles of RCTs to evaluate preventive interventions. The successes of RCTs in clinical medicine persuaded public-health researchers to use the technique to assess the health impact of health behaviors such as smoking cessation, condom use, consumption of fruits and vegetables, supplementations in vitamin and amino acids, and many other questions. Because these interventions were potentially good for health, they could acceptably be randomized.

In chapter 12, I discuss an issue illustrating the contribution of group comparisons to the establishment of health risks that has traditionally (and increasingly over time) attracted the attention and concern of epidemiologists: the relation of social inequalities to health. The example argues that social inequalities are responsible for about the same amount of premature deaths as tobacco (2011).

Chapter 12 also reports two examples of RCTs having prevention purposes. The Multiple Risk Factor Intervention Trial failed to show a benefit from a behavioral intervention in people at high risk of heart attacks (1982). The other example is the French study RCT SU.VI.MAX, which had an interesting and different conclusion regarding the still ongoing controversy about the ability of vitamin supplements to prevent cancer (2004).

Chapter 12 ends with an impressive success story: dietary transfatty acids, which in 1993 had been incriminated as harmful to the heart by the Nurses' Health Study, vanished twenty years later from the fast-food restaurant menus in New York City.

## IS THIS SCREENING USEFUL?

The involvement of epidemiology in the evaluation of screening programs was another indirect consequence of post-1945 technological and therapeutic progress: the availability of effective treatments and screening tests.

Before we see why epidemiology was instrumental in introducing a new way of determining whether screening for a particular disease was useful, please pause here and answer this question: When is it worth it to screen people for diseases? Or, rephrasing the question in a lengthier way: When is it worth it to indiscriminately propose to people belonging to a specific gender and age category a specific screening test to detect the presence of a disease in its earliest stages, before the person even feels sick and before a doctor can identify it with a clinical examination? Most of us have undergone screening tests in the past and still do. Why?

Studies have shown that few people, including doctors, understand that mass screening is worth it when screenees (on average, as a group) are likely to die at an older age from the detected disease than if they had not been screened.[16] Screening can be systematically offered only if it does help the screenees to live longer. Otherwise, it makes them uselessly aware of their ailment for a longer period of their life or, worse, submits them to the side effects of diagnostic procedures or avoidable treatments.[17]

The increased availability of effective treatments opened opportunities for screening. However, the habit of evaluating whether screening tests actually work is recent. Screening tests introduced before the 1960s were not evaluated. Doctors believed that the Bordet-Wasserman test for syphilis and the Papanicolau test for cancer of the uterus cervix worked, but there was no direct proof. These screening tests were easy to perform and to incorporate into the usual practice. This passive acceptance of screening changed in the early 1960s when an expensive and painful X-ray of the mammary gland, mammography, became available to screen for breast cancer: it was decided to determine first whether it prolonged life.

Chapter 13 discusses two RCTs of screening test efficacy: one that was deemed positive, suggesting that mammographic screening could prolong life (1963); another that was deemed negative, questioning the beneficial role of screening for the prostate-specific antigen to prolong the life of men suffering from prostate cancer (2009).

# 9

## IS THIS TREATMENT
## DANGEROUS FOR HEALTH?

### AMELIA AND THALIDOMIDE

"British Thalidomide Charity Rebuffs Gruenenthal Group's Apology" ran the headline.

> A British charity has rebuffed the first apology for half a century from the German company which invented birth defect pregnancy drug Thalidomide. The Gruenenthal Group said in a statement on its website that it "regrets" the consequences of the drug. Thalidomide was used to combat morning sickness but led to the birth of children without limbs during the 1950s and 1960s. Friday's apology was rejected as insufficient by the charity Thalidomide Agency UK, which represents people who were affected by the drug in Britain. Freddie Astbury, the charity's head consultant, said the company needed to "put their money where their mouth is" rather than simply express regret. Mr Astbury, who was born in Chester in 1959 with no arms and no legs after his mother took the drug, said: "If they are serious about admitting they are at fault and regret what happened they need to start helping those of us who were affected financially."[1]

Why did it take fifty years for Gruenenthal to apologize for having commercialized pills based on thalidomide since 1957? It has been estimated that these pills handicapped 40,000 adults and severely crippled 8,000 to 12,000 children worldwide. Half of these children died during their first year of life.[2]

This is the very dark story of scientific knowledge that a ruthless company tried to mask at the expense of the health of young mothers and their progeny. It started with the serendipitous discovery that pills containing thalidomide considerably reduced the feeling of nausea and the vomiting commonly affecting women during the first months of pregnancy. Sold over the counter, these pills came to be used as casually and abundantly as aspirin.[3] But their potential toxicity in humans had not been tested.

Let's focus here on how scientists were able to incriminate thalidomide in an epidemic of congenital malformation beginning in 1961. The pills had been on the market for about four years when William G. McBride, an Australian obstetrician, observed the unusual incidence of babies born amelic, without arms, legs, or other limbs, or phocomelic (which literally means "limbs of a seal"), with hands and feet but without arms or legs. He was under the impression that these babies had been delivered by mothers who had been given Distaval®, a drug containing thalidomide.

If McBride had asked for your advice, what suggestion would you have given him for a way to test his hypothesis that thalidomide was the culprit? Clearly, an RCT would not have been a good idea. This design is not an option for potentially harmful drugs. But a case–control study would have been appropriate: it would have allowed you to determine whether mothers of babies born suffering from amelia and phocomelia had used thalidomide during pregnancy more often than mothers whose children were born suffering from other forms of congenital malformations.

McBride used a different approach. He wrote to the editor of *The Lancet*: "In recent months I have observed that the incidence of multiple severe abnormalities in babies delivered of women who were given the drug thalidomide ('Distaval') during pregnancy, as an anti-emetic or as a sedative, to be almost 20%."[4] He regarded this percentage as extraordinarily high because in his experience congenital abnormalities were present in approximately 1.5 percent of babies.

Was this a group comparison? Formally, no. McBride only reported that 20 percent of the babies among the women to whom he had prescribed Distaval were malformed. He did not have a control group of women who had not used Distaval. But it was implicit that this control group comprised the rest of his practice: the frequency of abnormalities seen in the babies of thalidomide-consuming women was much higher than what he would have expected based on his experience with all the other women he followed during their pregnancy.

Thalidomide was not the first drug to have unexpected side effects, but the story was popularized by the lay press and quickly became a scandal. The drug was not authorized in the United States thanks to the scandal in Europe. Soon afterward, in 1962, the United States adopted the Drug Amendments to the Federal Food, Drug, and Cosmetic Act of 1938 and imposed the assessment of human risk before the commercialization of a new drug. Thus, it would have been more decent for Gruenenthal to apologize in 1962 than in 2012.

The thalidomide disaster modified policy with respect to pharmaceutical products, requiring proof of assessment of the risks for humans before the commercialization of a new drug. Epidemiologic group comparisons were one of the tools used in such assessments.

## DALKON SHIELD AND MYCOSES

The side effects of thalidomide were so dramatic that they could be identified without formal group comparisons. Fortunately, most drugs and medical devices usually have a less spectacular toxicity. Nevertheless, when in 1976 the potential harm caused by the Dalkon Shield, an intrauterine contraceptive device (IUD) first marketed nationwide in January 1971, came under the US government's purview, it had already caused several deaths. An IUD is a mechanical means of contraception. The presence of a foreign body in the uterus prevents the implantation of the fertilized egg. By June 1974, approximately 2.8 million units of this IUD had been implanted in women in the United States. It was initially suspected that because of the IUD's unusual shape, the process of removing it provoked later pregnancy complications. In the summer of 1974, the manufacturer voluntarily halted further distribution of the Dalkon Shield in the United States because of its reported association with pregnancy-related complications and in 1980 advised physicians to remove the Dalkon Shield even from asymptomatic women because of risk of infection.

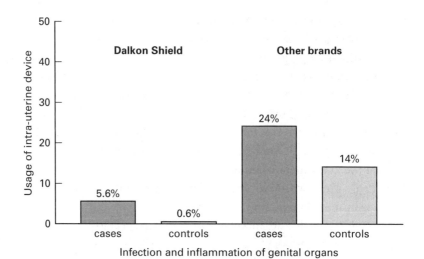

FIGURE 9.1 **Use of an Intrauterine Device (IUD) and Pelvic Inflammatory Disease**

Case–control study comparing usage of the Dalkon Shield IUD and usage of other types of IUD at the time of hospital admission among 622 women suffering from pelvic inflammatory diseases (cases) and 2,369 women free of pelvic inflammatory diseases (controls).

*Source*: Lee et al. 1983.

Here again, an RCT was not warranted. It would have been criminal to randomly allocate the Dalkon Shield or a different brand of IUD and compare the rates of pelvic infections. What would have been your optimal choice of study design? Because the number of women who used a Dalkon Shield and got a pelvic infection was expectedly small, a case–control study was a good fit to transform suspicions into evidence.

In 1983, a case–control study compared whether women hospitalized for an infection of the upper genital tract (i.e., the cases) had used the Dalkon Shield device more often than women hospitalized for other reasons (i.e., the controls).[5]

As shown in figure 9.1, only 5.6 percent of the cases had used the Dalkon Shield versus 0.6 percent of the controls, but this was nine times more (0.056/0.006 = 9.3) than the controls. For IUDs other than the Dalkon Shield, the relative difference was less impressive: 24 percent of the cases and 14 percent of the controls (0.24/0.14 = 1.7). Sales of the Dalkon Shield were eventually stopped.

## UNEXPECTED ADVERSE EFFECTS

Case–control studies have proved to be useful for identifying the unexpected adverse effects of medical treatments. They served, for example, to show that a hormone, diethylstilbestrol, used in the 1970s to prevent miscarriages, caused cancer of the vagina among daughters exposed in the womb; that oral contraception caused—in addition to heart attacks among smokers—deep venous thrombosis among women harboring the mutation of a genetic factor involved in the mechanism of blood coagulation (factor five—Leiden); that aspirin caused Reyes syndrome—a lethal coma—when prescribed to reduce flulike symptoms in children; that estrogen replacement therapy used during menopause caused breast cancer; and so on. All these adverse effects are rare, but these associations would probably never have been found without epidemiologic group comparisons.

Thus, group comparisons can be useful for identifying the adverse effects of medical treatments. There is, however, an important caveat: case–control or cohorts studies can be used for this purpose only if the doctors, when they prescribe the drug, have no clue that it can have that adverse effect.[6]

When doctors suspect a particular adverse effect, they avoid prescribing the treatment to people at high risk of suffering from the adverse effect. For example, they will avoid prescribing estrogen replacement therapy to women who smoke cigarettes because the combination of tobacco and estrogen-containing oral contraceptives has been shown to increase the risk of heart attack. Accordingly, if women receiving estrogen replacement therapy are at low risk of heart attack in the first place, a comparison with women not taking estrogen replacement therapy might fail to detect that the estrogen replacement therapy can cause heart attacks. In contrast, if doctors don't suspect the adverse effect, they prescribe the drug indiscriminately to all patients who may need it, and therefore if the treatment is toxic, a group comparison will show a higher frequency of the adverse effect among those receiving the treatment.

# 10

## DOES THE TREATMENT WORK?

### WHETTING TRIAL'S METHODOLOGY

It has taken about half a century to work out the practice of RCTs. Two main potential mistakes in their conduct were picked up from the early experiences.

In 1898 in Denmark, Johannes Fibiger, a twenty-eight-year-old physician, tested the efficacy of a serum containing antidiphtheria antibodies in treating patients suffering from diphtheria, a life-threatening form of sore throat. According to the day of hospital admission, patients suspected of having diphtheria were allocated to either the serum or no serum group. Only 8 patients out of 239 (3.3 percent) in the serum-treated group versus 30 out of 245 (12.2 percent) in the control group died, suggesting that the serum was effective. However, because the bacteriologic search for diphtheria took several days, Fibiger admitted the patients into the trial on the basis of only a clinical suspicion of the disease and later excluded from the trial those patients who were proved not to have diphtheria.[1] It seemed logical to remove from the trial people who did not have diphtheria and could not benefit from the expected therapeutic effect of the treatment anyway. Yet RCTs cannot suffer this kind of exclusion. Can you tell why? As randomized, the serum and nonserum groups could be expected to be comparable, but not necessarily after some patients were excluded secondarily. Note that this is true even when, as in this trial, the proportion of patients who were bacteriologically negative for bacteria was likely to have been randomized too and therefore similar in the serum and in the nonserum group. In the twentieth century, statisticians stressed that modifying group composition after randomization can jeopardize the group's comparability.

The second main form of mistake was identified in the 1930s in an English RCT that compared two treatments for pneumonia: a horse serum enriched in antipneumonia antibodies and bed rest.[2] Allocation of the two treatments was determined by the order of hospital admission: the first patient admitted for pneumonia received horse serum, the second bed rest, and so on. Serum seemed to reduce mortality among younger patients, but the researchers realized that the "alternate" method of allocation—one patient yes, one patient no—had a major methodological defect. Can you say what it was? The answer is not easy and was actually learned during the analysis of the trial results: doctors could easily guess the treatment of the subsequent patient. Driven by their clinical instinct, they did not always scrupulously respect the order of admission so that they could prescribe the horse serum preferentially to young patients who had a better prognosis. The benefit of randomizing was consequently lost, and the groups were not comparable anymore. The lesson was that a successful trial must conceal to the caregiver the allocation order of the experimental and control treatments.

By 1938, the lessons were learned. To protect the randomization, an American trial evaluating the prophylaxis of pertussis (whooping cough) vaccine concealed the allocation process and did not modify the groups after the randomization.[3] Concealment was done using a table of random numbers to decide the treatment allocation of two groups of children. This system of allocation used a list of completely independent numbers, half of them even and the other half odd. A number from the list was allocated to each child according to the order of the list: the first child in the list receiving the first number of the table, the second child receiving the following number, and so on. It might have been based on whether the random number was even or odd, but it was unpredictable by the vaccinators during the trial. The result was that 1,000 children received two doses of the vaccine, four weeks apart. They were compared to 1,000 nonvaccinated children. There were 51 cases of whooping cough in the vaccinated group and 150 in the unvaccinated group. The vaccine was deemed protective. Even though whooping cough was a major cause of childhood mortality, the results of this RCT did not seem to have immediate clinical consequences. It was not until the late 1950s that the pertussis vaccine was finally introduced on a large scale.

## TUBERCULOSIS, STREPTOMYCIN, AND ORWELL

Wider recognition of the importance of RCTs came from the first demonstration of the efficacy of a drug, streptomycin, against tuberculosis.

In the twentieth century, tuberculosis killed more people prematurely than cardiovascular diseases or cancer of any type. Although tuberculosis's mortality declined rapidly between 1850 and 1948, it started from much higher levels than other diseases. In 1900 in Europe and in the United States, annual mortality rates were often greater than one per thousand.[4] Tuberculous patients were commonly treated in everyday medical practices. The discovery of an effective treatment would have impressed both the doctors and the general public.

In 1943, streptomycin, an antibiotic produced by a fungus, like penicillin, was shown to be effective against the Koch bacillus, the tuberculosis-causing bacteria, first in the test tube and then in tuberculous guinea pigs. It was, however, deemed very expensive by the newly created English National Health Service—hence, the idea to test whether it was effective in humans before providing it to doctors. An RCT was the natural choice.

In the trial, tuberculous patients were randomized either to treatment with streptomycin or to bed rest.[5] The randomization procedure was equivalent to shuffling a deck of cards and prescribing streptomycin if a red card was drawn or bed rest if a black card was drawn. The one addition was that envelopes containing the group allocation were ordered in such a way that the content was unpredictable—that is, "concealed" from the researchers. Before the admission of a patient into the streptomycin trial, the appropriate numbered envelope was opened at the central office; the card inside revealed if the patient was to receive streptomycin or not. This information was then transferred to the medical officer at the center. Thus, learning the lessons of the past, this RCT incorporated sound techniques for both randomizing the treatment and concealing from the doctors the order in which the streptomycin was allocated.

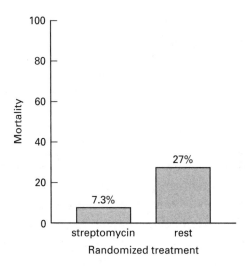

FIGURE 10.1  **Risk of Death from Tuberculosis, 1948**

Risk of death by tuberculosis over six months (percentage) in the streptomycin RCT conducted in England in 1948.

*Source*: Medical Research Council 1948.

What health benefit was observed? The two grams per day of streptomycin that were given intramuscularly at six-hour intervals proved to be effective (figure 10.1). During the first six months, there were four deaths among fifty-five patients (7.3 percent) allocated to streptomycin, compared with fourteen deaths among fifty-two patients (27 percent) allocated to bed rest alone. The difference was impressive.

In this RCT, one group of patients received a course of streptomycin, whereas the other was restricted to bed rest and no pharmaceutical treatments. Because the groups were properly randomized, they can be expected to have been, on average, very similar in terms of age, severity of the disease, and factors other than their allocated treatment.

This 1948 streptomycin trial was a milestone victory against a disease that had been a major public-health enemy for centuries.[6] For the first time, an antibiotic proved to be capable of killing the bacteria responsible for tuberculosis.

The trial had a limitation, however. Do you see what its flaw was?

The control group was assigned only to bed rest. It did not receive some form of medication too. Optimally, it should have received intramuscular injections, four times per day, of a serum that had an identical appearance as the streptomycin injections but wasn't streptomycin. Both groups would have been equally fooled by the expectations they placed in streptomycin. This heavy regimen's only purpose, however, would have been to balance the design of the study. Moreover, streptomycin had violent adverse effects that would make patients receiving it realize that they were not on a placebo. The British novelist George Orwell wrote in his last notebook a lucid and poignant description of his suffering because of streptomycin, a treatment that he had to prematurely interrupt:

At first, though the streptomycin seemed to produce an almost immediate improvement in my health, there were no secondary symptoms, except that a sort of discoloration appeared at the base of my fingers & toe nails. Then my face became noticeably redder & the skin had a tendency to flake off, & a sort of rash appeared all over my body, especially down my back. There was no itching associated with this. After about 3 weeks I got a severe sore throat, which did not go away & was not affected by sucking penicillin lozenges. It was very painful to swallow & I had to have a special diet for some weeks. There was now ulceration with blisters in my throat & in the insides of my cheeks, & the blood kept coming up into little blisters on my lips. At night these burst & bled considerably, so that in the morning my lips were always stuck together with blood & I had to bathe them before I could open my mouth. Meanwhile my nails had disintegrated at the roots & the disintegration grew, as it were, up the nail, new nails forming beneath meanwhile. My hair began to come out, & one or two patches of quite white hair appeared at the back (previously it was only speckled with grey).

After 50 days the streptomycin, which had been injected at the rate of 1 gramme a day, was discontinued. The lips etc. healed almost immediately & the rash went away, though not quite so promptly. My hair stopped coming out & went back to its normal colour, though I think with more grey in it than before. The old nails ended by dropping out altogether, & some months after leaving hospital I had only ragged tips, which kept splitting, to the new nails. Some of the toenails did not drop out. Even now my nails are not normal. They are much more corrugated than before, & a great deal thinner, with a constant tendency to split if I do not keep them very short. At that time the Board of Trade would not give import permits for streptomycin, except to a few hospitals for experimental purposes. One had to get hold of it by some kind of wire-pulling. It cost £1 a gramme, plus 60% Purchase Tax. [7]

Thus, the absence of a placebo in the streptomycin trial was probably a minor limitation because of streptomycin's terrible adverse effects.

## "I WILL PLEASE" (IN LATIN)

In some way, it became established that the impact of a treatment depended not only on the active substance it contained, but also on the medical care provided, the caregiver–patient relationship, the empathy toward the patient, and the patient's belief in its effectiveness. The potential benefit of these extra factors was dubbed the "placebo effect." [8]

The word *placebo* is the first-person, future tense of the Latin verb *placer*. It means "I will please." How did the term end up in the jargon of RCTs? I am not sure. One explanation goes like this: Prayers by priests at funerals in the Middle Ages began with the word *placebo*, "I will please." Those in poverty had to pay for these prayers when they lost a relative or a friend. This was an expense for the living, but was it really useful to them or to the dead? Over time, the term *placebo* became synonymous with "useless action," and, with this sense, it entered the jargon of RCTs.

A placebo is—most of the time, but not always—an inactive substance that looks exactly like the real drug. As a rule, participants agree to be unaware of whether they will receive the active treatment or the placebo, but they all expect to be taken care of equivalently. Indeed, RCTs should not be conducted when there exists evidence that the experimental treatment works better than the placebo. Yes, placebos do please. It was already observed in the 1950s and 1960s that they were effective. Here are some early examples. [9]

In the 1950s, it was hypothesized that tying off the mammary arteries that run behind the breastbone would increase the flow of oxygen to the heart muscle in patients suffering from what still has the antiquated name "angina pectoris." This Latin name for coronary heart disease means "a strangling feeling in the chest" because such is the feeling when the heart muscle begins to lack oxygen. Surprising as it may be, at the time some surgeons believed that the vascular system worked as a network of rigid tubes and that interrupting the blood flow in one tube would increase it in the other tubes. They hoped that by tying off the mammary artery, they would increase the pressure in the heart (coronary) arteries and thus prevent the crisis of angina pain from occurring when the patients exercised. A study carried out at the University of Kansas Medical Center with twenty-three subjects consisted of comparing mammary artery ligation with a placebo surgery. For the placebo surgery, a surgeon made an incision in the skin but did not tie off the artery. Thus, both groups of patients woke up with similar scars on their chests, but members of one group had the mammary artery tied off, and members of the other group did not. When asked about their symptoms afterward, all five patients who had the placebo surgery (100 percent) claimed they had improved, could exercise more, needed less drugs, and felt well, compared to only 75 percent of the eighteen subjects whose arteries were tied off.[10] In other words, the placebo surgery had "worked" better than the arterial tie-off. Arterial ligation surgery is no longer performed.

The next example of a placebo effect is the key to success for any practicing physician. It involved randomizing the message doctors gave to patients who had been seen for generic symptoms and turned out not to have any organic ailments. Half of the patients were given a diagnosis and told that they would be better in a few days. The other half was told that "the doctor could not be sure what was wrong." Both groups were comparable. Two-thirds (64 percent) of the patients who received the positive message improved versus only 39 percent of those who received the more unpromising message. Reassuring words from a doctor helped, without any treatment attached.

Although we do not understand the placebo effect's exact biological mechanisms, these examples illustrate real placebo effects in treating pain and in treating subjective problems—such as "feeling better."[11] In a synthesis of thirty-four RCTs of drug treatments for depression, placebo alone produced an improvement of the depressive state equivalent to 75 percent of the improvement obtained using antidepressive drugs. If the group receiving the experimental treatment had an average score of 10 on a depression scale, the score in the placebo group was between 7 and 8.[12] However, interventions that have objective outcomes—such as quitting smoking, for example—seem to have little or no placebo effects.

## AZT, AIDS, AND DISCORD

Ideally in an RCT, thanks to randomization, the groups to be compared should be very similar. Yet is this still true if during the phase of observation following randomization some patients quit the study, stop taking the randomized treatment, or adopt the treatment of the group they have not been randomized to? Would you still consider the remaining groups interchangeable? Did I hear you say, "Yes, because I assume that all the changes occurred randomly"? This assumption would be audaciously hopeful, however. In practice, those who quit or switch treatment are likely to be different from those who remain in the study and comply with their therapeutic regimen. Group comparability may suffer badly from postrandomization shuffling of group composition.

To maintain the initial group comparability despite subsequent losses and dropouts, the rule of RCTs is to analyze the participants according to the treatment with which the investigator had intended to treat them. This "intention to treat" principle is founded on keeping subjects in their original groups even if, in practice, they did not receive the prescribed treatment. For example, participants who had to take treatment A but in reality took treatment B will be analyzed as if they had taken treatment A even though they did not. At first, this approach sounds counterintuitive, but it makes sense if you remember that the fundamental difference between an RCT and another study design is the randomization of the subjects. This is the one thing you want to preserve.

Consider the situation in which treatment switches are so common that by the end of the trial about half of the participants in each of the compared groups took the experimental drug. Would you be willing to accept the verdict of the analysis under the intention-to-treat rule? There is no easy answer to that question, but these were more or less the terms of the controversy that surrounded the interpretation of the RCT named

"Concorde" that was conducted between 1988 and 1992 in France, England, and Ireland.[13]

The Concorde study tested against placebo the efficacy of azidothymidine (AZT), then a new drug meant to fight HIV. People who had been infected with HIV would typically after some period of time become clinically ill and develop AIDS. Concorde tested whether AZT could slow down this evolution. Therefore, all participants were seropositive for HIV but were not yet showing any clinical symptoms of AIDS. One group received AZT immediately, whereas the other received a placebo, which was to be replaced by AZT as soon as they developed any clinical signs of AIDS.

Was this a group comparison? Yes, it was an RCT.

Which groups were compared? HIV-seropositive subjects treated immediately with AZT or subjects first given a placebo, which was to be replaced by AZT as soon as they developed clinical signs of AIDS.

How much health benefit was observed? In the final analysis of the trial, the risk progression to AIDS was 18 percent in both groups (see figure 10.2). This progression corresponded to a zero percent risk reduction. There was no expectation of delaying the progression to AIDS by using AZT.

There was, however, a source of concern. Patients allocated to the placebo were immediately aware that they did not suffer from the known AZT side effects such as anemia and abdominal pain or headaches and faintness. Among them, 37 percent requested to be prescribed AZT and started taking it earlier than they should have according to the initial study protocol. Thus, large fractions of both groups had received AZT early. What would you have done? Many believed that the trial was flawed because an effect of AZT could have been artificially diluted. There remained the option of comparing those who had actually received AZT early with those who did not, independently of the group in which they had been randomized. Was this an acceptable second-best option? Unfortunately not. This analysis would not have been based on the exchangeable groups generated by randomization. The benefit of having performed an RCT would have been lost. The nonrandomized analysis can be done, but its findings cannot be claimed as resulting from an RCT. A benefit of AZT could have been due to another trait conferring a better prognosis to those who took AZT.

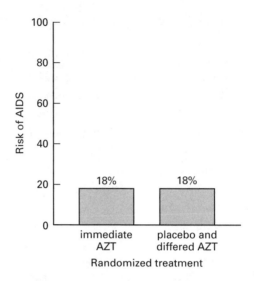

FIGURE 10.2 **Progression Risk to AIDS or Death, 1988–1992**

Three-year risk of progression to AIDS according to immediate AZT treatment or placebo followed by AZT in the Concorde RCT. The analysis is based on whether patients had been allocated to one group or the other ("intention to treat"), not on whether they had actually taken AZT or the placebo.

*Source*: Concorde Coordinating Committee 1994.

Today we know that the Concorde study, despite all its imperfections, led to the correct conclusion: AZT alone does not slow down the progression of AIDS. But in 1994, in the socially and politically tense climate surrounding issues related to AIDS treatment, its results were received with more skepticism than they deserved because of the methodological problems mentioned here.

# 11

# WHAT IS THE OPTIMAL
# MEDICAL DECISION?

## A TOSS-UP FOR PULMONARY EMBOLISM

Consider a hypothetical clinician in the 1960s who suspects a young patient of having a "pulmonary embolism," an acute disease of the lung. Excruciating pain occurs when a bullet made of a fibrous protein and blood cells, called an "embolus," clogs a vessel that normally provides blood to a region of the lungs. Lacking oxygen, the lung tissue does not function properly, and the patient cannot breathe anymore. Depending on where in the lung an embolism occurs, the patient may feel pain, shortness of breath, or die from sudden suffocation due to lack of oxygen. Pulmonary embolism is a difficult disease to diagnose because many diseases of the heart, the gut, and the pancreas can produce similar clinical symptoms. It is, however, critical to make a rapid and accurate diagnosis because pulmonary embolism is a lethal disease if not timely treated.

Our doctor requests a newly available diagnostic procedure for her patient, an angiography, which consists of injecting in the blood a product that has the ability to strongly absorb X-rays. The product enters the heart and is expelled into the vessels leading to the lungs. When the product reaches the lungs, an X-ray is taken, which provides a detailed, bright molding of the lung vascular tree over a dark background. If some blood vessels are obstructed by an embolus, they will typically look as if they have been cut off, an image that is extremely rare to see in the absence of a pulmonary embolism.

Unfortunately, in this example, the angiography itself causes a lethal hemorrhage. Having learned from this experience that angiography is a dangerous procedure, the clinician is leery to use it again and immediately prescribes a drug treatment to the next patient she suspects has a pulmonary embolism. The doctor is aware that the drugs may be prescribed in vain if the patient ends up not having a pulmonary embolism, but at least the patient will be spared the risk of undergoing an angiography. The drugs that effectively treat pulmonary embolism block the coagulation process that caused the embolus and may aid in dissolving it. These anticoagulants have to be prescribed for several weeks.

Unfortunately again, the anticoagulated patient is inadvertently injured and dies of a hemorrhage. Now, having learned from this second experience, the clinician becomes leery of using anticoagulants too, and she neither immediately prescribes anticoagulants for nor subjects to angiography her next young patient suspected of having a pulmonary embolism. This decision is also risky because one out of three untreated pulmonary embolisms is fatal.

Without needing to say what happens to the third patient, the key point of this saga is that a single doctor's experiences are not sufficient for recommending one form of medical management over another for a patient suspected of having a pulmonary embolism. However, the risks associated with angiography, anticoagulants, or no treatment and the proportion of tests that return false positive or false negative results can be measured in populations of patients. This is why in the 1970s a small group of clinicians invented "clinical decision analysis."

In the previous example, the clinician is faced with three options: prescribe anticoagulants immediately; perform an angiography and prescribe anticoagulants if that test confirms the pulmonary embolism; or wait, without prescribing either treatment or angiography. Clinical decision analysis can help identify the "optimal" care for a given patient suspected of having pulmonary embolism.

There is no guarantee that the "optimal" decision will save a particular patient, but it is the option that has the greatest chance of success if the clinical decision analysis is based on the appropriate data. With colleagues in Geneva, I tried to adapt clinical decision analysis to the bedside management of pulmonary embolism in emergency wards. We summarized the analysis in a graph, allowing the doctor to choose rapidly the optimal decision according to the clinical probability of pulmonary embolism and the result of a noninvasive test.[1] The graph stimulated physicians to make accurate clinical observations and reduced the usage of invasive diagnostic procedures such as angiography.

## LET'S EBM TOGETHER

CAPRISA 004 was an RCT on the efficacy of a vaginal gel containing 1 percent tenofovir in preventing HIV infections among sexually active women.[2] It was conducted in Kwazulu-Natal, South Africa, between 2007 and 2010. The US Centers for Disease Control and Prevention rightly announced that the results were "an exciting step forward for HIV prevention": "Women represent the majority of new HIV infections globally, and urgently need methods they can control to protect themselves from infection. It is also very encouraging that the study found that the microbicide significantly reduced the risk of genital herpes (HSV-2), which is common in developing countries and in the United States, and facilitates HIV transmission."[3]

The 889 trial participants were HIV-negative women ages eighteen to forty who had engaged in vaginal sex at least twice in the thirty days prior to screening. They were randomly assigned in equal proportions to either tenofovir gel or placebo gel. Both gels appeared identical, were dispensed in the same prefilled vaginal applicators with identical packaging, and had to be used following the same intercourse-related strategy: one dose of gel to be inserted within twelve hours before sex and a second dose of gel as soon as possible within twelve hours after sex.

At the end of the study, the infection rate was 5.6 percent per year among the group using the tenofovir gel and 9.1 percent among those using the placebo gel (figure 11.1).

Was this a group comparison? Yes, it was an RCT.

Which groups were compared? South African women allocated either to a group receiving a vaginal gel containing tenofovir or to a group receiving a placebo vaginal gel.

How much health benefit was there? This is where EBM chimes in. Let's EBM together.

We can begin by subtracting the infection rates to compute the rate difference:

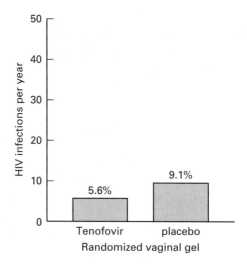

FIGURE 11.1 **HIV Infection Incidence Rate, 2007–2010**

Risk of HIV infection according to use of a vaginal gel containing tenofovir or a placebo vaginal gel in the CAPRISA 004 RCT, conducted in Kwazulu-Natal, South Africa, between 2007 and 2010.

*Source*: Karim et al. 2010.

Rate difference = infection rate in the placebo group minus the infection rate in the tenofovir group = 9.1 – 5.6 = 3.5% per year.

What does the rate difference mean? The placebo group had an excess rate of HIV infection of 3.5 per 100 women per year. This also means that the tenofovir gel prevents 3.5 HIV infections in 100 women who use it for a year.

There is, however, a different way to express the rate difference, which is very neat. In EBM, it is referred to as the "number needed to treat" to prevent one health event, abbreviated NNT. It is an interesting way of reformulating the question about the trial results. The rate difference directly answers the question "How many HIV infections can be prevented for 100 women using the gel before and after sexual intercourses for a year?" The answer is 3.5 infections can be prevented. The question can be reformulated as "How many women need to be treated for a year in order to prevent one infection?" Now the answer is 29.[4] Proportionately, it is the same thing: treating 100 women to prevent 3.5 HIV infections is equivalent to treating 29 women to prevent one infection.[5] But many people, including me, find the NNT more telling of the efficacy of the treatment than the rate difference. An NNT of 29 is low, indicating that the tenofovir gel is very effective. It is easy to perceive that, applied to the millions of HIV-negative women who become sexually active each year, the gel can make a difference.

Thus, twenty-nine women need to use the anti-HIV gel before and after sexual intercourse during one year to avoid one of them getting infected. Unfortunately, the NNT is rarely reported in the media, which prefer to report how much more risk or less risk is associated with a treatment. Most newspaper articles about CAPRISA 004 said that the gel "gave women a 39 percent chance of avoiding infection." Where does the 39 percent come from?

In EBM jargon, it is the relative rate reduction (RRR), obtained by dividing the infection rate difference by the infection rate in the placebo group:

RRR = rate difference ÷ rate in the placebo group
    = (9.1 − 5.6)/9.1 = 0.39, or 39%.

The interpretation of the RRR is that the tenofovir gel is associated with a 39 percent HIV-infection rate reduction compared to the rate in the placebo group. The RRR is commonsensical. We easily recognize a reduction of 10 percent, 30 percent, 50 percent, and so on.

Thus, in the CAPRISA 004 RCT, a full EBM summary of the answer to the question "How much health benefit was observed?" reads that the HIV infection rate was 5.6 percent per year when a vaginal gel containing tenofovir was used before and after sexual intercourse, which corresponds to a 39 percent RRR for the tenofovir users compared to the women using the placebo gel. This treatment has the expectation of preventing one HIV infection for every twenty-nine women who use the tenofovir gel for one year.

# 12

# HEALTH RISK OR HEALTH BENEFIT?

## DOES EDUCATION DETERMINE WHO LIVES AND WHO DIES?

An 2011 *New York Times* article titled "Researchers Link Deaths to Social Ills" stated the following:

Poverty is often cited as contributing to poor health. Now, in an unusual approach, researchers have calculated how many people poverty kills and presented their findings, along with an argument that social factors can cause death the same way that behavior like smoking cigarettes does. . . .

The researchers used various criteria to define an adverse social condition. Low education, for example, was defined as not having graduated from high school. Poverty was defined as a household income of less than $10,000. A population in which more than 25 percent of people reported their race or ethnicity as non-Hispanic black was considered racially segregated. The study also calculated the effect of an area's overall poverty level, income differential and low social support.

For 2000, the study attributed 176,000 deaths to racial segregation and 133,000 to individual poverty. The numbers are substantial. For example, looking at direct causes of death, 119,000 people in the United States die from accidents each year, and 156,000 from lung cancer.

Social factors are not the same as diseases or accidents, but Dr. Galea argues that they are equivalent to a behavior like smoking, and that, as with smoking, there is evidence of the mechanism involved. . . .

"If they had not smoked, 400,000 people each year would not have died," Dr. Galea said. Similarly, he said, if they had graduated from high school, the 245,000 people whose cause of death he attributes to low education would still be alive.

Was this a group comparison? Yes, because in order to attribute a number of excess deaths to any of these social factors, one needs to compare those exposed with those unexposed to that factor. The social factors analyzed in the original publication are low education, poverty, lack of health insurance, employment status, occupational stress, lack of social support, being victim of racism or discrimination, poor housing conditions, stress during early childhood, living in areas that are poor and in a deteriorated built environment, racial segregation, high crime and violence, low social capital, and absence of open or green spaces.[1]

Which groups were compared? For low education, the mortality in people who did not graduate from high school is compared with the mortality of people having at least a high school diploma or equivalent; for income, a household with an annual income of less than $10,000—that is, below the poverty level—is compared with households above that level; or for area poverty level, the excess mortality of people living in areas in which 20 percent or more of the population lives below poverty level is compared with the mortality of people living in areas where less than 20 percent live below the poverty level.

How much health harm was observed? The newspaper article mentions that there were 176,000 excess deaths due to racial segregation, 133,000 excess deaths due to individual poverty, and 245,000 excess deaths (a quarter of a million) due to low education.

How did Dr. Sandro Galea and his colleagues technically compute these excess numbers of deaths? A simple way to summarize what they did is to view these excess numbers of deaths as a series of multiplications:

Percentage of excess mortality attributable to a characteristics (A) × percentage of the US population with a given characteristic (B) × total number of deaths (C) = excess number of deaths in people with the characteristics(D).

The percentage of excess mortality (A) is derived from group comparisons. Take, for example, low education in Americans ages twenty-five to sixty-four years old. Dividing the mortality rate of people with low education (less than a high school diploma) by the mortality rate of the rest of the US population yields a rate ratio of 1.8, corresponding to a percentage of excess mortality of 80 percent.[2] Census data indicate that 16 percent of the US population is without a high school diploma (B). National mortality statistics indicate that in 2000 one million deaths occurred (C). Thus, the excess number of deaths attributable to low education in this age group is:

A × B × C = 80% × 16% × 1 million = 128,000 deaths.

This difference of 128,000 deaths is equivalent to saying that 564,000 deaths occurred in people with low education versus 436,000 in the rest of the population ages twenty-five to sixty-four years old.

How many excess deaths were attributable to low education among those age sixty-five years or older given that the mortality rate ratio is 1.2, the prevalence of low education is 34.5 percent, and the number of deaths 1,800,000?[3] Do you get 124,200 excess deaths? Altogether, low education may cause 252,200 deaths (128,000 + 124,200). This is a little bit more than the 245,000 deaths the original publication found using a more complicated formula, but the point here is to realize that the rate ratio, derived from a group comparison is at the core of this finding.

## MISTER FIT

In 1970, the Multiple Risk Factor Intervention Trial, or MRFIT (pronounced "Mister Fit"), had ambitious and captivating goals. It was designed to test the efficacy of a prevention program against coronary artery disease (obstruction of the arteries that irrigate the heart by atherosclerosis).[4] It aimed to assess the impact in the general population of what had become the standard medical advice given to middle-aged men at high risk of coronary artery disease: reduce dietary fat and high cholesterol, stop tobacco use, control hypertension, and so on.

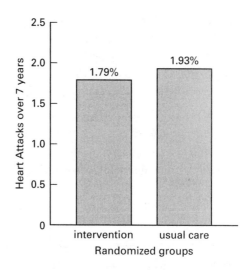

FIGURE 12.1 **Risk of Heart Attack Over Seven Years, 1972–1982**

Risk of death from coronary artery disease over seven years in 12,866 men (6,428 in the group that received the multiple risk factor intervention and 6,438 in the group that had the usual care) in the US Multiple Risk Factor Intervention Trial (MRFIT). The mortality risk was of the same order of magnitude for both groups: about 2 percent.

*Source*: Multiple Risk Factor Intervention Trial Research Group 1982.

The trial lasted seven years, from 1974 to 1981. The 12,866 participants, all men ages thirty-five to fifty-seven at high risk of coronary artery disease, were selected from 361,662 men examined in twenty-two US clinical centers: 6,428 men received the intervention, and 6,438 others were sent to their usual doctor with a report listing the values of their risk factors. The participants in the intervention group were motivated and informed. For all these years, they had to be ready, as needed, to stop smoking, be treated for hypertension, and go to a clinic regularly, sometimes with their family.

MRFIT had cost $180 million by 1980. It was an expensive attempt to persuade people to change their lifestyle and improve their risk profile. The results after 10.5 years showed a small benefit to the intervention (see figure 12.1).[5] The reasons for the unexpectedly modest effect of prevention are still debated today. Maybe the press coverage of the benefits expected from the intervention led people in the comparison group also to engage in preventive behaviors, hoping to benefit from them. Or maybe the interventions were not able to transform the participants' daily lives beyond the trends observable in the US society as a whole: men in the United States were quitting smoking, and hypertension was being treated at a much larger scale, anyway. My personal opinion is that more attention should have been paid to actively involving the communities in the design and implementation of interventions that aimed to modify their daily lives.

## DO THIRTEEN ORANGES A DAY
## KEEP CANCER AWAY?

Diet lends itself well to RCTs, but it has also proved to be a perilous area of study. Think of vitamins. These almost mythical molecules are widely perceived as having only benefits. The industries producing them have achieved the prowess to advertise them as if they belonged to complementary and alternative medicine, when in reality they are pharmaceutical products.

The principle of isolating a molecule, concentrating it, and using megadoses of it against a virus (e.g., influenza) or a cancerous cell is typical of industrialized allopathic medicine. Consider the recommendation of taking 1,000 milligrams of vitamin C during the winter season to prevent the flu. Our bodies can absorb such a dose of vitamin C only after overcoming their natural defense against intoxication. Our feeling of satiety, which took at least tens of millions of years to evolve, would warn us against eating thirteen oranges at a sitting, each containing 80 milligrams of vitamin C, in order to meet the 1,000-milligram prescription. And the recommendation can be achieved only by using refined vitamins concentrated into pills or powder—that is, a pharmaceutical product. I doubt that bypassing our natural defenses to ingest a vitamin "bomb" in order to destroy a virus or a cancerous cell is truly compatible with mainstream canons of holistic medicine.

The hype surrounding vitamins soon extended to cancer therapy. Two-time Nobel laureate Linus Pauling promoted his belief that high doses of vitamin C could keep cancer away. There was no evidence supporting that belief then, and there is still none today. But a strong case could be made in the 1980s that beta-carotene, a precursor of vitamin A, was protective against cancer. The theory sounded plausible. Beta-carotene can neutralize molecules that can bind with DNA in the cell nucleus and induce mutations capable of transforming a normal cell into a cancerous one. Moreover—and here epidemiology failed—comparative cohort studies leaning in that direction abounded.

Therefore, still in the 1980s, researchers in Finland and the United States tested against a placebo the prescription of massive doses of beta-carotene to prevent lung cancer among heavy smokers. The results of these RCTs were stunning. High doses of beta-carotene did not protect against cancer; instead, they may have been even more dangerous than the placebo according to two of three of the trials.[6]

How could science have erred this much? The biology of beta-carotene indicates that it should be protective against lung cancer. Cohort studies suggested that its consumption was associated with a lower risk of cancer.

Why do you think the results of the RCTs and cohort studies could have diverged so much?

A French RCT launched in 1994, SU.VI.MAX—which, after translation, stands for "Supplementation in Antioxidant Vitamins and Minerals"— offered a plausible explanation. Its underlying idea was that the effect of high doses of vitamins may be different from the effect of small doses found in a balanced and healthy diet. SU.VI.MAX was therefore designed to test whether doses considered optimal for the human body, from a physiologic point of view, could be protective against cancers and other noncommunicable diseases.

A total of 13,017 French people (7,876 women and 5,141 men), ages forty-five to sixty, were randomized to receive either a capsule cocktail of low doses of vitamins C, E, and beta-carotene and the antioxidant minerals selenium and zinc[7] or a placebo capsule. They were selected out of 79,976 volunteers and followed for seven and a half years. Minitel, the French ancestor of the Internet, was used to record treatment compliance and occurrence of health events.

How much heath benefit was observed? Figure 12.2 shows that in men the seven-year risk of cancer was 3.5 percent in the experimental group and 4.9 percent in the placebo group.

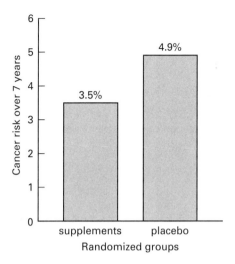

FIGURE 12.2 **Cancer Risk and Use of Supplements Over Seven Years**

Seven-year risk of cancer in French men ages forty-five to sixty, randomized to receive either a capsule cocktail of vitamins C, E, and beta-carotene and the antioxidant minerals selenium and zinc or a placebo starting in 1994–1995 in the SU.VI.MAX study.

*Source*: Hercberg et al. 2004.

Let's answer this question, once again, the EBM way. In the SU.VI.MAX RCT, the seven-year risk of cancer among men was 3.5 percent in the experimental group, which corresponds to a risk difference of 1.4 percent compared to the group who received the placebo and to the expectation of preventing one extra cancer for every seventy-two men receiving the vitamin and antioxidant supplementation for seven years.

In women, vitamin supplementation did not impact cancer risk. Female participants started the trial already with higher dietary levels of beta-carotene than men as a result of a higher consumption of fruits and vegetables. They did not need to be supplemented as much as the men, and for this reason they probably did not benefit from additional antioxidants.

The main lesson of SU.VI.MAX is that providing an antioxidant supplementation equivalent to that found in a healthy diet does not increase cancer risk. It may even reduce risk in people who are nutrient deficient. A second conclusion is that a balanced diet rich in fresh fruits and vegetables does not need to be supplemented by vitamin pills at all. Incidentally, that a balanced diet keeps cancer away sounds much more consistent with a holistic approach than the concentrated thirteen-orange pills.

Even though the beliefs about the miracle effects of antioxidant vitamins such as beta-carotene, vitamin C, and vitamin E remain very prevalent, the knowledge accrued over the past twenty years actually indicates that megadoses of beta-carotene and vitamin E can be toxic and shorten one's life expectancy.[8]

## TRUE NURSES, ARTIFICIAL TRANSFATS, AND NEW YORK CITY RESTAURANTS

What can French fries, microwave popcorns, frozen pizzas, baked goods, margarines and spreads, ready-to-use frosting, and coffee creamers have in common? They can contain "transfatty acids," nicknamed "transfats"—that is, solid fat artificially made out of liquid oil mixed with hydrogen. Hydrogenation straightens out the normally kinked fat molecules and changes their metabolic properties, making them stable for deep frying (e.g., the French fries emerge from the fryer crisp and yellow, not brown). Food manufactured with transfats has a long shelf life. Industrial transfats are economically attractive but not indispensable. Some healthful fatty acids have similar properties.

In the early 1990s, many believed that industrial "transfats," particularly because of their straight shape, akin to that of saturated fats, could get deposited in the arteries and cause heart attacks. Evidence, however, was lacking to support these beliefs.

What type of study design would you opt for to study the association of transfat and heart attacks? You preferably would assesses the dietary habits current at a time when none of the participants has suffered from heart attacks. It is difficult for healthy people to remember what they used to eat five or ten-year ago, but memory is even less faithful when a disease or its treatment have caused food aversion or profound modifications of dietary habits. Contrasting the past diet of people who have suffered heart attacks with that of people who have not—that is, a case–control study—is therefore not optimal to solve the transfat enigma. A cohort study comparing the occurrence of heart attacks among high and low consumers of transfat is appropriate, but it needs to be large: even in a population at high risk of heart attacks, less than a dozen events can be expected to occur per 1,000 people and per year. Assessing the food content in transfats is also challenging because they contribute to about 2 percent of Americans' caloric intake. The dietary assessment needs to be rigorous to reckon the variability in transfat in the population. In other words, you want a large cohort study able to measure diet accurately in tens of thousands of people, right? Indeed, the Nurses' Health Study was this type of luxurious design that lent itself to test the health effects of transfat consumption.

The Nurses' Health Study began in 1976, when 121,700 US female registered nurses completed questionnaires about their health and health-related habits. The nurses were then contacted every two years to update their information and report new diagnoses of major illnesses. Beginning in 1980, an additional questionnaire began to assess their dietary habits. New techniques, used in education to scan school tests, made it possible to process 100,000 detailed questionnaires every two years. Notably, participants faithfully adhered to the study since its inception. The Harvard team behind the original Nurses' Health Study successfully competed for hard-to-get funds from the National Institutes of Health to prolong the study for more than thirty years and enrich it with second and third studies and a cohort comprising the original participants' children.

In 1993, a first analysis of the 431 heart attacks observed among 85,085 nurses over eight years indicated that a difference of three grams in daily intake of transfat increased the risk of coronary heart disease by 30 percent.[9] This was a cohort study. The groups compared differed by the amount of transfat in their diet. The rate of coronary heart disease (per thousand and per year) were 0.6 for a daily intake of 2.4 grams of transfat and 0.8 for an intake of 5.7 grams. The ratio of these two rates, 1.3 (0.8/0.6), translates into a 30 percent increased risk of coronary heart disease between the extreme categories of transfat consumption. The connection was weak, but several other cohort and case–control studies, involving 142,000 subjects and 6,200 coronary heart events, subsequently confirmed that a difference of two to three grams of transfat increased the risk of coronary heart disease by 29 percent![10]

A remarkable chain of administrative and legal decisions transformed the epidemiologic finding into public-health policy. In 2003, ten years after the Nurses' Health Study report, the Food and Drug Administration required labels of manufactured food to indicate the amount of transfat. Check any US food label. The listed amount of transfat is likely to be 0 gram or zero percent per serving. The Dietary Guidelines for Americans and the Institute of Medicine further recommended that individuals keep trans-fatty acids consumption as low as possible.

In 2006, New York City restricted restaurants from using, storing, or serving food that contained more than a minimal amount of transfats. The regulation became fully effective by July 2008. Its impact was evaluated by the New York City Department of Health.[11] In 2007 (before the regulation) and in 2009, the purchases made by 15,000 clients from 168 fast-food restaurants selling mostly hamburgers, sandwiches, fried and grilled chicken, Mexican food, and pizza were compared. The transfat content per meal had dropped from 2.91 grams in 2007 to 0.51 grams in 2009. The 2.4 gram difference is of the same order of magnitude as that between the extreme categories of the Nurses' Health Study. Impressively, the reduction in transfat was not compensated by an increase in unhealthy saturated fat.

Thus, twenty years after the first epidemiologic alert, many heart attacks are prevented in New York City. Converting epidemiologic discoveries into effective policy is a relatively slow process, but stakes are high: avoiding transfat across the United States can, according to the Centers for Disease Control, prevent 10,000 to 20,000 heart attacks and 3,000 to 7,000 coronary heart disease deaths each year.[12]

# IS THIS SCREENING USEFUL?

## MAMMOGRAPHY AND BREAST CANCER

An RCT was launched in 1963 among women covered by the Health Insurance Plan of Greater New York (HIP).[1] HIP was—and still is—a prepaid insurance plan covering the care provided by doctors belonging to the plan. In 1963, there were 62,200 women, ages forty to sixty-three, who had belonged to HIP for at least one year. After randomization into two groups,[2] the 31,000 women of the experimental group were invited to get a regular mammographic screening plus breast examination, but nothing was changed in the usual care of the other 31,000 women who composed the comparison group. When breast cancer was suspected on the mammogram, a small amount of cells or tissues was collected from the mammary gland and examined microscopically. If cancer was found in this "biopsy" sample, the affected breast was fully removed along with the lymph nodes of the adjacent armpit. HIP facilitated the follow-up of all female members.

In this New York study, mammography performed at regular intervals (e.g., every two years) reduced mortality from breast cancer, particularly among women ages fifty to sixty-three.

Was this a group comparison? Yes, it was an RCT.

Which groups were compared? Groups were composed of women who belonged to HIP. Half of the women were prescribed regular mammographic screening plus breast examination, and the other half received the usual care.

How much health benefit was observed? After seven years of follow-up, the mortality risk difference was small for women ages forty to forty-nine

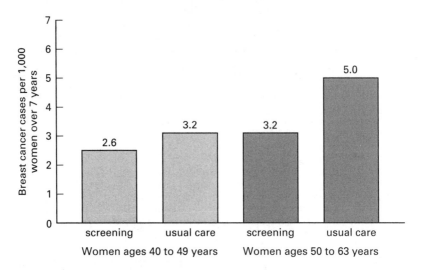

FIGURE 13.1  **Risk of Death from Breast Cancer Over Seven Years, 1963–1970**

Results of the New York Health Insurance Plan study, which began in 1963: risk of breast cancer after seven years of follow-up according to whether the participants in the RCT received regular mammographic screening or not and according to the age of the participants at the beginning of the trial. There were 29,760 women ages forty to forty-nine, of whom 14,849 were randomized to the screening group, and 32,240 women ages fifty to sixty-three, of whom 16,151 were randomized to the screening group.

*Source*: Gøtzsche and Nielsen 2009.

(2.6 and 3.2 per 1,000), but more substantial for women ages fifty to sixty-three (3.2 and 5.0 per 1,000), as shown in figure 13.1.

You may think that I am getting inconsistent here. I said the objective of screening is to prolong life, but here I conclude that the HIP trial indicated that mammographic screening of women fifty to sixty-three years old worked because the screening group has a lower mortality rate. Actually, mortality and longevity are two sides of the same coin: dying less from a disease means that one lives longer with it. Consider a screening test reducing mortality by 10 percent per year. The test would theoretically increase life expectancy by 10 years (100 years/10). What would be the number of years of life gained if the mortality rate among women age fifty were 1.2 percent per year in the screened group and 1.3 percent per year in the nonscreened group?[3]

There have been, since the HIP study, several other RCTs of mammographic breast cancer screening in Scandinavia, the former Soviet Union, Canada, and England. Not all of these trials confirmed the results of the New York study. The question of knowing whether mammographic screening helps or not, especially for women before the age of fifty, is still fiercely debated.[4] Mammographic screening may have prevented deaths from invasive breast cancer because effective treatments were made available to cases with early cancer detection. Today, the inverse question is raised. Does the combination of available effective treatments—adjuvant chemotherapy and hormonotherapy for cancers at stage 2 or beyond—and screening by clinical or self breast examination make mammographic screening obsolete? The answer to this question lies in the interpretation of existing data by the experts. There are currently no plans to launch any new RCTs on the issue.

## PSA AND PROSTATE CANCER

Now let's consider the screening for prostate cancer.

There is a blood test that detects a protein known as "prostate-specific antigen," or PSA. The test is benign and relatively inexpensive. PSA tends to be elevated in the presence of prostate cancer and low in the absence of cancer. Interpreting the test results is unfortunately not so simple, however, because PSA can also be elevated in the absence of cancer and can be low despite cancer. In short, PSA does not suffice to diagnose prostate cancer.

In practice, when PSA is low, men are told that they have no cancer, and no further investigations will be made until the test is repeated one year later. But if PSA is high, it is necessary to confirm the presence of cancer by collecting prostate cells. These cells are obtained by inserting a needle several times into the prostate through the perineum or the rectum. Prostate cells can then be examined with a microscope to confirm or rule out cancer.

RCTs have been conducted to determine whether PSA screening performed at regular intervals permits an earlier diagnosis and, on average, prolongs the duration of the life of men by preventing death from prostate cancer or at least by postponing it. In 2009, results of two of these trials were released. One was conducted in the United States and the other in Europe. The studies randomly allocated men older than fifty-five to either a group given regular PSA testing or to a group not tested regularly. The members of the two compared groups had very similar health profiles. The results were disappointing. Screening identified prostate cancer more often but did not reduce cancer deaths and prolong life duration compared to the no-screening control group.[5] Moreover, negative side effects of treatment, such as sexual impotence, were more common in the screened group.

The PSA test is currently a poor screening tool. It can lead to potentially useless major surgery capable of ruining many men's sexual life. Why is this so? First, the test itself does not discriminate neatly the presence of prostate cancer from its absence.[6] And second, it is more likely this type of screening will detect slow-evolving cancers, which often do not represent a life threat. The bottom line is that, in its present form, screening for prostate cancer using the PSA test does not make death from prostate cancer occur at an older age, although many urologists and oncologists find this conclusion too extreme.[7]

## OTHER SCREENING TESTS

Among the screening tests assessed using RCTs, besides mammography for breast cancer and the PSA test for prostate cancer, I can mention the following: for colon cancer, detection of blood in the feces (effective) and direct visioning of the gut walls and biopsy using optic fibers devices (effective); and for lung cancer, chest X-ray (ineffective) and CT scans (effective among heavy smokers).[8]

# 14

---

# GROUP COMPARISONS ALSO FAIL

THE PREVIOUS chapters have provided examples of dramatic situations in which epidemiology contributed to replacing beliefs with knowledge. Digressing throughout the book about the errors that can plague group comparisons would have obscured the message about the positive function of epidemiology. I have sketched, however, an overly confident profile of the discipline and of what it can deliver.

If I confess now that group comparisons can fail, would you be surprised? I did mention, for example, that cohort studies had long been interpreted as evidence of vitamin A's protective effect on some cancers. All sciences can fail, but this is no excuse for lenience: the issue of faulty group comparisons deserves serious attention. Epidemiology is a population science, and its failures can potentially affect many people at once. In September 2004, when rofecoxib (Vioxx), a nonsteroidal anti-inflammatory drug causing heart attacks was withdrawn from the market, it had been prescribed to an estimated 80 million people. It had taken four years, eleven RCTs involving 14,200 participants, 44 heart attacks to observe its adverse effect, and four more years to ban the drug.[1]

Let's review two examples of group comparisons that failed for different reasons: the cause of Kaposi's sarcoma and the effects of hormone replacement therapy on the heart. In these health issues, group comparisons first erred. Nevertheless, in contrast to what would have happened if we had been misguided by beliefs, beneficial lessons were drawn from these failures. It was possible to understand what went wrong and learn how not to repeat the same mistakes. These errors provided an objective basis for a critical debate. Despite the mistakes and sometimes the considerable human drama, they contributed to knowledge.

## POPPERS AND KAPOSI'S SARCOMA

In April 1981, I was in my third year of training as a medical doctor in Geneva. I had been taught that Kaposi's sarcoma was a slow-evolving skin cancer seen mostly in Africa. All of a sudden, though, several cases of Kaposi's sarcoma were identified among young gay men in the United States. The US cases differed from the textbook description in that they had a rapid and fatal evolution.[2]

It was first speculated that an infection, a food, or a drug could depress these patients' immunologic response and provoke the rapid clinical progression. But the mystery proved harder to solve than expected. Eight months later, in December 1981, while new cases arose, several competing hypotheses about the origin of this new form of Kaposi's sarcoma were still being debated, such as a combination of viral infection, drugs, and genetic predisposition; corticoid creams; sperm instilled in the rectum; amyl nitrite (a substance sold under the street name "poppers" and used particularly for its enhancing properties during anal intercourse); and a very large number of sexual partners.

At this stage, what would you have suggested as the method of choice to determine whether one of these hypotheses was correct? A few dozen cases had been diagnosed in the United States, and there was no dominant clue as to whether the disease had a chemical, infectious, or immunologic origin.

For the rare event with such a varied list of potential causes, a case–control study was the most realistic choice of methodology: the cases were patients diagnosed with Kaposi's sarcoma; the controls were people without Kaposi's sarcoma. The delicate step was in the choice of controls. To be comparable to the cases, controls had to have lived similar lives as the cases but to have remained free of Kaposi's sarcoma. The comparison should reveal a factor that the cases were exposed to, but not the controls. Asking, measuring, and comparing past exposure to chemical, infectious, and immunodepressing factors provided an opportunity to test each of the candidate causes and identify those for which there was a difference between the cases and the controls.

Indeed, that same year, 1981, a case–control study was conducted among homosexual men in New York.[3] A cluster of twenty patients diagnosed with Kaposi's sarcoma was identified at New York University Medical Center. Two homosexual controls of the same race and age were chosen for each case from the practice population of a Manhattan physician, most of whose patients were homosexual men. The two main findings about people with Kaposi's sarcoma were that they were twelve times more likely to have had 542 experiences or more with poppers (versus less than 542 experiences) and twice as likely to have had ten or more sexual partners per month (versus less than ten). The interpretation of the results, after weighing the pros and cons of each hypothesis, leaned toward incriminating poppers (a chemical cause) rather than the number of sexual partners (an infectious, potentially transmissible cause).

One year after the publication of the case–control study, in May 1983, a great discovery made the front pages of newspapers around the world: the AIDS virus, a T-lymphotropic retrovirus, had been isolated.[4] Was Kaposi's sarcoma caused by the same virus? The available data were reconsidered under this new perspective. It was first thought that the AIDS virus discovered in 1983, later baptized "HIV," was the culprit. In August 1983, epidemiologists declared that "the variables most strongly associated with Kaposi's sarcoma or pneumocystis pneumonia [are] those related to [the] number of sexual partners and meeting such partners in bathhouses."[5] But some patients with Kaposi's sarcoma, including one case in the case–control study discussed earlier, had never been infected with HIV. It took several years to find out that a sexually transmitted herpes virus was involved in the causation of Kaposi's sarcoma.[6]

It would be ludicrous to criticize today the errors that were made in the heat of a threatening epidemic. On the contrary, those who reacted, performed studies, and generated data must be commended for having done the right thing at the right moment. Unfortunately, an opportunity had been missed to insist on the sexually transmitted nature of the disease for at least a year before the discovery of HIV. As long as no precise cause was forthcoming from the laboratories, epidemiology remained on the frontline. Instead, incorrect ideas were propagated about the cancer-provoking role of poppers. This example might make you think that epidemiology is not reliable. What went wrong? Why were poppers seriously considered as the culprit instead of simply as a marker of sexual activity?

## INCOMPARABILITY AND CONFUSION

The example of poppers and Kaposi's sarcoma is a case in point of group incomparability, an issue of fundamental importance for the design and interpretation of group comparisons. I did not discuss group incomparability in the previous chapters for the sake of simplicity, but it was dealt with in all the historical examples we have reviewed.

The most intuitive way of visualizing group incomparability is to consider a cohort study in which each group is a mix of people harboring characteristics that put them at different risk of the studied outcome. Say you have identified a group of dog owners and another of cat owners, and you count the heart attacks that occur in the two owner groups over the following ten years. Your hypothesis is that owning dogs protects against heart attacks because it incites more physical activity than cat ownership. Each group can be split in two subgroups: people younger than age fifty, and people fifty years or older. The subgroup age fifty plus is on average at higher risk of heart attack only because of its age. Clearly, if 75 percent of the dog owners are age fifty and older versus only 20 percent of the cat owners, the two groups are incomparable: dog owners will a priori suffer more heart attacks than cat owners. The difference may be unrelated to dog ownership and strictly due to the difference in age. It would be inappropriate to rapidly conclude that your hypothesis was wrong: because of the incomparability in age, the effect of dog ownership, if any, and the effect of age on heart attacks are confused, or—in epidemiologic jargon—confounded. A valid comparison requires that the two groups have the same proportion of people age fifty or older.

Incomparability in age is easy to suspect and would be taken care of in the analysis of any group comparison. The typical expression for taking care of it is that the comparison is "adjusted" for age. Because prominent group incomparability has rarely escaped the scrutiny of researchers and the experts who evaluated their work, teachers of epidemiology often rely on hypothetical examples as I did with the cat and dog owner study to demonstrate the mechanisms of the phenomenon. But the case–control study of poppers and Kaposi's sarcoma is one of the rare historical examples in which a group incomparability went unnoticed and had serious consequences.[7]

Underlying every case–control study, there are real-life cohorts evolving in the community. In a case–control study, group incomparability does not refer to the case group versus the control group, who are expected to be different, but on the exposed versus unexposed members of the underlying cohorts who later become cases or not. In our hypothetical example of dog ownership and heart attacks, replace dog ownership with popper consumption (less than versus more than 542 experiences); age with number of sexual partners (less than versus more than ten per month); and heart attacks with Kaposi's sarcoma. The discovery of a viral origin of Kaposi's sarcoma made it clear that more sexual partners meant more exposure to sexually transmitted viruses. Heavy popper consumers spuriously appeared to be at increased risk of Kaposi's sarcoma because they comprised a greater proportion of highly sexually active men than did the moderate consumers. A proper interpretation of the study, however, should have emphasized the sexual transmissibility of the agent causing Kaposi's sarcoma rather than the extreme consumption of poppers.

In retrospect, we can wonder why it was not immediately obvious that the number of poppers consumed was a close correlate to the number of times engaged in sexual intercourse. For example, gay men formed only one of the communities in which cases of Kaposi's sarcoma had been diagnosed; cases from other populations (e.g., intravenous drug users, hemophiliacs, and heterosexuals) did not use poppers, at least not in the same order of magnitude.[8]

The mistake that was made in the investigation of Kaposi's sarcoma also reflects the intrinsic difficulty of assessing group incomparability: there is no objective criterion for deciding when groups are comparable and when they are not. At some point, it is a subjective decision and, as such, can be influenced by our lack of emotional neutrality. Sometimes wrong expectations may interfere with our interpretation of what the data reveal. I discuss this point more thoroughly in the last section of chapter 16. We approach epidemiological results with a mind that is not neutral toward any interpretation, but that is loaded with beliefs, opinions, expectations, past experiences, biases, and so on. In 1982, the researchers who studied Kaposi's sarcoma may have been influenced by the piling up of examples of detrimental chemical products, such as the tragedy of thalidomide. If the chemical substance contained in poppers was the culprit, the epidemic of Kaposi's sarcoma could be stopped by rapidly and universally dropping poppers as an aphrodisiac. The context may have mattered, too: the magnitude of the mounting epidemic was still unpredictable, in particular among heterosexuals, but focusing on a high number of sexual partners as the culprit would have stigmatized some communities more than others.

## HORMONES, ETERNAL FEMININITY, AND BROKEN HEARTS

"At any age, you can be FEMININE FOREVER. The documented story of one of medicine's most revolutionary developments and breakthroughs— the realization that menopause is a hormone deficiency and totally preventable. Now, almost every woman, regardless of age, can safely live a full sex life for her entire life."[9]

This book blurb on *Feminine Forever* by Robert Wilson uses all the traits of a fad: total satisfaction and safety guaranteed to "almost every woman." This New York gynecologist promised that hormonal pills could "prevent" menopause and sustain youth, beauty, and sex "forever."

The rationale was simple and seductive. A lower secretion of ovarian hormones—estrogen and progesterone—after menopause produced, around age fifty, hot flashes, mood swings, sleep disturbances, and other unpleasant symptoms. It could be counteracted by a newly available pharmacological substitution for the normal secretion of ovarian hormones, called "hormone replacement therapy." In 1949, Premarin was the first commercialized replacement estrogen. It seemed to boost cancer of the uterus, however, whereas Provera, a replacement for progesterone, reduced the risk of that same cancer —hence, the idea of combining estrogens and progesterone into one drug named "Prempro," a contraction of the first syllables of the names "Premarin" and "Provera."

For Wilson, Provera would attenuate or even eliminate the unpleasant symptoms of menopause without incurring cancer risks. Here is an example of the form of logic he used to promote the universal usage of estrogen replacement therapy from age thirty on:

> As this is being written, in late 1965, I have just completed an intensive study of eighty-two cases in which menopause was effectively prevented or cured by the use of estrogenic birth control pills. The women in my research group ranged from thirty-two to fifty-seven years with an average of 45.8 years. The study represents a total of 132 patient-years and 1591 menstrual cycles. Of twenty-seven patients who took birth control pills specifically to avoid menopause, twenty six were completely successful. They never developed any menopausal symptoms. The single exception experienced only mild symptoms. The other patients in this group took birth control pills to relieve menopausal symptoms that had already set in. This proved effective in ninety-three percent of these cases. . . . In the study of eighty-two patients just cited, not a single case of systemic, breast, or genital cancer was observed. Much more significant is the report presented in 1964 by Drs. Gregory Pincus and Celso Ramon Garcia to the International Union Against Cancer. Their study comprised 5,374 cases of women using contraceptive tablets. None of these women developed cervical cancers after starting the use of the pills—an incidence far below the normal statistical cancer expectancy.[10]

Where is the error in this reasoning? Wilson took a small group of selected patients, found absolutely no failures, and generalized his findings to all women in the world. There was no comparison. We know by now that—except for unusually dramatic effects—group comparison is indispensable to draw conclusions about the effectiveness or the safety of a drug therapy. His study would have been much more informative had he at least randomized the replacement therapy.

However, complexity mounted in the story when nonrandomized comparative cohort studies found that women on Prempro had a lower risk of heart attacks in addition to attenuated menopausal symptoms and osteoporosis. These same studies also indicated that the risk of breast cancer increased. Then again, as a balance, the excess number of breast cancer cases seemed small compared to the number of prevented heart attacks and bone fractures.

Proclamations about the virtues of hormone replacement were so compelling that the US National Institutes of Health hesitated to submit its efficacy to rigorous testing. Large fractions of menopausal women were already being given hormone substitutes. It was believed that these women were slashing their heart disease risk by half. Would you have considered it ethical to take away such a miracle drug from thousands of women in a comparison group to determine whether the postulated benefits were just hype or not? This was a tough decision to make, but hormone replacement had become so prevalent that its health impact needed to be rigorously evaluated. The National Institutes of Health finally opted for the Women's Health Initiative, an RCT.[11]

In this RCT, menopausal US women still with a uterus were randomized to take either estrogen plus progestin[12] replacement therapy or a placebo. The rate of developing coronary artery disease was 0.37 percent per year in the hormone replacement group and 0.30 percent in the placebo group (figure 14.1).

How much heart benefit was observed? Let's answer this question, once again, the EBM way now that we are familiar with it. In the Woman's Health Initiative RCT, the rate of developing coronary artery disease was 0.37 percent per year in the hormone replacement group and 0.30 percent in the placebo group. For the hormonally replaced group, there was a rate in excess of 0.07 percent per year compared to the group who got the placebo. I invite you to compute the NNT to provoke one extra heart attack. What did you get?[13] Indeed, the Woman's Health Initiative indicated that hormone replacement therapy provoked one *extra* death from coronary artery disease for each 1,429 women receiving the treatment for a full year. Of note, the number 1,429 is sometimes referred to as the "number needed to harm" rather than the "number needed to treat." Hormone replacement caused more heart attacks than the placebo!

The Woman's Health Initiative RCT found the opposite of what Wilson claimed and nonrandomized group comparisons had suggested. Instead of being cut in half, the risk of coronary artery disease was greater among women receiving the hormone replacement therapy than among those receiving the placebo.

Women and the medical community were flabbergasted by the results. Hormone replacement therapy was extremely popular. As an example of

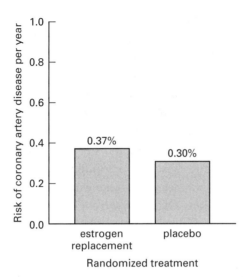

FIGURE 14.1  **Annual Risk of Death from Coronary Artery Disease**
**and Estrogen Replacement Therapy**

Annual risk of coronary artery disease according to whether the participants, menopausal American women with a uterus, were randomized to take estrogen replacement therapy or a placebo.

*Source*: Rossouw et al. 2002.

a population for which we have data and which was probably not atypical of a Western nation, in 2002, just before the publication of the Woman's Health Initiative results, hormone replacement therapy was prescribed to half of the menopausal women in Geneva. One year after the results were published, only 31 percent of these menopausal women were still being given this treatment—that is, about the same proportion as in 1993, before the great infatuation with hormone replacement.[14]

## WHEN RESULTS CONFLICT

Why did the cohort studies and the RCT yield conflicting results? Which one could be trusted? An attractive hypothesis was proposed after it was observed that there were two periods during which hormone replacement increases cardiovascular risk: during the first twenty-four months of treatment and when treatment began more than ten years after menopause.[15] These two risk periods were not equally distributed in the RCT and in the nonrandomized cohort studies. Here is why.

Participants in the Woman's Health Initiative were different from the "typical patients" for whom the treatment is meant to be eventually prescribed. Patients with atypical symptoms or poor prognosis, those who are difficult to track, and those who are unlikely to comply with the prescribed regimen were not included, with the intention of guaranteeing the trial's technical conditions. Of the 373,092 eligible women, only 16,608 (4.4 percent) women were deemed eligible and accepted to participate in the trial. The selected women had to be willing to receive either replacement hormones or a placebo without knowing which of the two they would receive. Therefore, women who had already been receiving the hormone replacement for many years were also less likely to be included in the study. Why should they risk depriving themselves of a treatment they were happy with?

The participants also belonged to an age group in which coronary artery disease was not too rare. The mean age of the participants was sixty-three years, resulting in about half of them being already menopausal for more than ten years when they started the first twenty-four months of replacement therapy. Participants thus accumulated the traits of a group at high risk for having heart problems under hormone replacement therapy: their first two years of hormone replacement occurred ten years or more after menopause. The increased risk of heart attack observed in the RCT may be valid only for women whose first hormone substitution occurs ten years or more after menopause.

In contrast, the typical women in the nonrandomized cohort studies had just reached menopause. They could have received the treatment for two years or more and were therefore beyond the high-risk time window (first twenty-four months of treatment). The women who had suffered heart problems while under therapy most likely stopped their treatment. Women who had had a heart attack after initiating therapy but *before* completing the cohort study questionnaire had to be excluded from the analysis. Thus, the women under therapy, however long they had been treated, were likely to be at low risk of heart disease, whereas the women who were not under replacement therapy were likely to have been at high risk of heart disease.

The way participants had been selected into the cohort study resulted in a spuriously large proportion of women at low risk of heart disease among the current users of hormone replacement therapy. The group comparison suggested that hormone replacement therapy was protective against coronary artery disease when it was not. Any suggestion regarding how this source of bias could have been avoided? Had the cohort studies restricted the comparison to newly treated women with never-treated women, they might have been able to identify the transitory increase in coronary artery disease risk during the first two years of replacement therapy.

The debate about the harmlessness of hormone replacement therapy is still ongoing,[16] but new RCTs that have learned from past trials and consider the high-risk time periods in their study design will accrue new knowledge. Robert Wilson's claim of eternal femininity was merely a belief. We did not learn much from disproving the "feminine forever" concept except to distrust its author. In contrast, as epidemiologists Robert Hoover and Jan Vandenbroucke stress, we have learned from the failed cohort studies: the discussions to reconcile or explain the apparent differences between the cohort studies and the RCT have improved epidemiology's methods, enlightened our knowledge about how and when hormone replacement therapy can be prescribed, and further elucidated the causes of coronary heart disease.[17]

# 15

## EPIDEMIOLOGIC LITERACY AND
## "EARTHLY SELF-REALIZATION"

THE YEAR 2013 marked the two hundredth anniversary of the birth of John Snow, the London anesthesiologist who had the brilliant idea to compare the clients of two water companies in order to prove his hunch that the polluted water of the Thames, as was popularly believed, was responsible for the humongous cholera outbreaks of 1854 (see chapter 4).

Many reasons motivate epidemiologists to celebrate this achievement. Snow did not form his beliefs solely by chance: all sorts of evidence had already convinced him that cholera was a contagious disease. He was therefore prepared to seize the exceptional opportunity to determine whether the clients of a water company having moved its pumps to a clean place of the Thames would suffer less from cholera than those of the company that kept pumping its water in the center of London. He (personally) collected a mass of data, counted, compared, discovered what we know today as the right conclusion, and invited society to act. He incarnates a model epidemiologist.

The celebration in 2013 facilitated the opportunity to raise a question that has agitated the US Institute of Medicine[1] and other similar institutions for many years now: When will epidemiology be integrated into the school curricula? One of the articles in a series published in *The Lancet* for that occasion stated: "Given the power of epidemiological methods in the assessment of human experience and endeavor, and its implicit role in so many discussions and decisions at the core of the everyday lives of all people, one might ask whether the subject should now be introduced as an obligatory part of the general science curriculum in secondary schools. We think so."[2]

I think so, too. Note that the goal of epidemiologic literacy mentioned in this quotation would be to empower citizens for decision making at "the core of the[ir] everyday [life]." Indeed, the present time is opportune for generalizing basic epidemiology education. Current public trends demand it. There is an abundant search for health information on the Web. Roughly half of all adults between the ages of eighteen and sixty-four used the Internet to search for health information in 2009, according to a six-month study conducted by the US Centers for Disease Control and Prevention. Internet searches for health-related websites is such a common practice that they may even serve as sensitive indicators of emerging epidemics, a phenomenon National Public Radio has called "webidemiology."[3] Millions of people simultaneously entering the same health-related keywords in their search engines may raise a flag before the cause of their concerns manifests into cases seen in emergency rooms and medical offices. This is a profound, international, new, and positive phenomenon: the emergence of an educated public that is thirsty for health knowledge.

How would understanding the principles of group comparisons change the way people search for health information on the Web? People would know how to separate knowledge from the mass of personal beliefs, opinions, and other unsupported theories that often bury accurate health knowledge.[4] Moreover, a tremendous amount of anxiety and many unsafe decisions might be avoided.

However, as we have learned from our review of the history of epidemiology, there is an additional portentous reason for teaching epidemiology: there seems to be no other way to acquire its principles than by learning them. Thus, acquiring those principles is dependent on the incorporation of epidemiology into the formal school curriculum.

We have seen that it has taken a significant amount of time (at least 4,000 years) and scores of lost lives for society to develop a science of epidemics. It took an additional 350 years, since 1662, for medicine and public health to embrace epidemiology. Clearly, the union formed among society, epidemiology, and the latter's methods did not happen in an instantaneous "Eureka!" moment. It was an arduous process.

Even now that epidemiology has a presence in universities and in the media, not many people are familiar with it. Epidemiology is infamously arcane, even though, as this book shows, there is no intrinsic complexity to it. On the contrary, the principle of comparing groups of people involves no more than simple logic. Thus, we can wonder why people didn't rely on group comparisons to support the practice of medicine and public health before the end of the seventeenth century? Why did it take additional centuries for society to internalize epidemiology's methods, and why is familiarity with epidemiology still so uncommon?

Here is a plausible explanation: thinking in terms of populations is something human psychology struggles with. Apparently, no one spontaneously acquires the notion that risks are an attribute of populations and not individuals and that some health questions have exact answers for populations, but not for the individual. As stressed several times in this book, there does not seem to be a common life experience that teaches us the fundamental difference between an individual who is unique and whose health trajectory is unpredictable and a population or group of people whose health evolution can be predicted and compared. There is no historical evidence that population thinking is a skill acquired during the normal growth of intelligence. It takes some education. Pioneers of the discipline acquired it through self-learning. Reading the original prose of John Graunt (chapter 3), John Snow (chapter 4), Pierre Louis (chapter 5), and Adolphe Quetelet (chapter 4), to name only a few early population health scientists, reveals the elation engendered by their unexpected discovery of the regularity and predictability of traits in populations. The advantage today is that we can formally learn the concepts elucidated in this book from the lessons amassed by society over the past 350 years. The obstacle human beings face in becoming population thinkers might explain both the late genesis of epidemiology and society's slow acquaintance with it. This struggle is manifest in history, and it is obvious in classrooms.

Thus, to acquaint citizens with epidemiology, there seems to be no alternative than to teach epidemiology in middle and high schools, colleges, and universities as part of the basic education, along with public speaking, writing, math, and other sciences. It would also be possible, realistic, useful, and timely to integrate epidemiology into continuing education courses for adults. The outcome would be epidemiologic literacy, which will allow citizens to access and evaluate the explosion of health information available in mainstream publications.

## HUMANS OR LANGUISHING GODS

Population thinking is—in my view—the most difficult concept that teachers have to transmit and students need to acquire. Population thinking is the most intellectually challenging component of epidemiology because it involves concepts, such as the concept of risk, valid for populations and not for individuals. Students have to learn to move back and forth between two universes governed by different rules. It is like learning to evolve in a fifth dimension when our familiar world has only four (see chapter 1). Once this skill is acquired, the principles of group comparisons come naturally.

Risks are measured in populations. Consider (the realistic) lifetime risks of lung cancer as being 10 percent among ever smokers versus 0.5 percent among never smokers. These risks are tangible in a population of say 200 people: out of 200 lifelong smokers of at least one pack per day, 20 will get lung cancer; out of 200 lifelong never smokers, one will get lung cancer. But for an individual these risks are mere abstractions: we cannot say which individuals—John, Janet, Pierre, or Wade—will develop lung cancer over a period of time.

This abstraction makes epidemiology seem like an imprecise science, providing only half of an answer. A 10 percent lifetime risk is enormous, but it is not 100 percent. A 0.5 percent risk is much smaller, but it is not zero percent. For individuals, only certainties make immediate sense: "If I smoke, I will get lung cancer. If I do not smoke, I will not." In practice, these certainties do not exist.

Errors of reasoning occur when the distinction between the two universes, that of the individual and that of the population, becomes blurred, when the difference between a 100 percent risk and a 10 percent risk is not properly interpreted. For example, I can think, "If I smoke, I will get cancer," but the proper interpretation of the 10 percent risk is: "If I smoke, I most likely will not get lung cancer." Similarly, it is inappropriate to equate a 0.5 percent risk among never smokers to a zero percent risk. I think, "If I don't smoke, I will not get cancer," but the proper interpretation is, "If I don't smoke, I am unlikely to get lung cancer."

This confusion happens all the time. Take for example the 2011 press release disseminated by many media claiming that "fatty fish" may cut risk of an eye disease called "macular degeneration." You can, as I did,

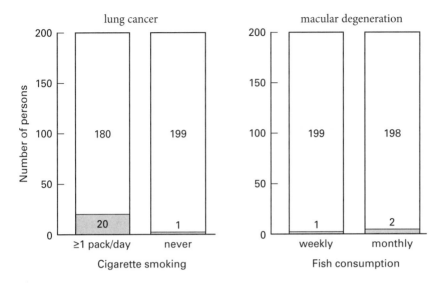

FIGURE 15.1 **Lifetime Risks of Lung Cancer
and Ten-Year Risk of Macular Degeneration**

Numbers of cases (*gray*) and noncases (*white*) of lung cancer or of ocular macular degeneration that are expected in a population of 200 individuals according to the categories "cigarette smoking" (*left*) and "fatty fish consumption" (*right*).

*Sources*: Doll and Hill 1964; Christen et al. 2011.

informally inquire about people's reactions to it. Most of those who take the information seriously conclude that if they eat one or more servings of fish per week they will not get age-related macular degeneration. Others discard the information as implausible. Originally, the fatty fish–macular degeneration association is health knowledge. Misinterpreted, it becomes a belief.

For an accurate interpretation of health risks, it can help to project ourselves as a unit of a population. As a unit in a population of 200 smokers (see figure 15.1), if I smoke a pack per day, I might be among the 20 (10 percent) who will get lung cancer, or I might be among the 180 who will not. If I don't smoke, I can be the one who will get lung cancer in the group of 200 never smokers (0.5 percent) or among the 199 who will not. Ten percent and 0.5 percent are the population risks. I can subtract them and see that in the population smokers have 9.5 more percentage risk points of getting lung cancer than never smokers. This health knowledge can inform my individual decisions and help me choose whether to act, if this is within my wheelhouse, or to ignore it.

If you now apply the same reasoning to the risk of ocular macular degeneration, the interpretation of group comparisons to inform your individual choices should become even more evident. By looking further into the original scientific publication,[5] you can learn that the ten-year risk is 0.5 percent for those who eat one or more servings of fish per week and 1 percent for those who eat less than one serving of fish per month. As a unit of a population of 200 people who eat fish weekly, I might be the one who will develop the eye disease over the next ten years, or I might be among the 199 who will not. If I eat fish less than once per month, I can be among the two who will get eye disease or among the 198 who will not. In the population, weekly fish eaters have 0.5 less percentage risk points for developing macular degeneration over ten years than the less than monthly eaters of fish. The intentionally inconspicuous difference between the dark sections of the two rectangles on the right of figure 15.1 is meant to translate graphically how difficult it can be to make sense of tiny risks for individuals. In comparison, the risk among smokers is huge.

Thus, risks are attributes of populations, not of individuals. Still, comparing risks can inform individuals about potential developments in their every day life.

At first, population thinking is painful and demands practice. But once we become used to transitioning from the individual to the population level and vice versa, population thinking can be really cool.

For students who will still complain that they are not interested in uncertain knowledge, we can encourage them to consider the opinion of the novelist, playwright, and philosopher Jean-Paul Sartre, who held uncertainty as an essential characteristic of the human condition: "Living implies short-term prediction and coping as best as we can. Maybe our fathers, with a little bit more science, could have understood that there was no solution to a given problem, that a question was poorly stated. But the human condition requires that we make blind choices: there is no morality without ignorance. If we knew all the factors that determine specific phenomena, if we were always sure to win, not only would risk vanish, but also courage and fear, expectation, final joy and effort; we would be languishing gods but not humans."[6]

Wouldn't this be a great topic for a student essay in an epi class? Epidemiology gives us access to a form of knowledge that may not be exact, but that is compatible with our human condition. It can inform our choices but not determine them.

## TEACHING IN SCHOOLS

In 1987, the epidemiologist David W. Fraser stressed that epidemiology was a "low-technology" science readily accessible to nonspecialists, applicable to a broad range of interesting phenomena, emphasizing methods rather than arcane knowledge, and combining "the scientific method, analogic thinking, deductive reasoning, problem solving within constraints, and concern for aesthetic values."[7]

He elegantly linked scientific method, problem solving, and aesthetics in a way that neither Sherlock Holmes nor Albert Einstein would refute.

The main question at this point is to choose an angle that makes epidemiology attractive to students. One option, as I have done in this book, is to take advantage of contextual aspects that can grasp the attention of even middle school students. The long voyages and naval battles of the ships of the Royal Navy were propitious for scurvy and James Lind's trial (chapter 3). The epidemics of cholera investigated by Snow highlight the drinking-water crises that crippled bulging metropolises (chapter 4). Ignaz Semmelweis's tale puts the slow evolution of obstetrics in perspective at a time when giving birth was a major life threat (chapter 5). The life of cotton mill workers in small villages and of sharecroppers in the old cotton fields of South Carolina is the backdrop of Joseph Goldberger's elucidation of the link between poor diet and pellagra (chapter 6). And so on. Each of these tales remarkably addresses the main threats to people's health in the past. The solutions to these threats required courage, creativity, and the use of detective skills.[8]

In high schools and (European) lyceums, it is possible to add some quantitative concepts such as risks, risk differences, and risk ratios to discuss health examples relevant to teenage life. The key questions to ask students are: "How do we know . . . ?" and "How can we know . . . ?" How do we know that contraception is safe, tobacco harms, addiction affects cognitive development, condoms protect against sexually transmitted diseases? How can we know whether usage of cell phones and laptop computers can impact health? The answers to all these questions invariably involve carrying out group comparisons such as those discussed in this book. Examples of group comparisons provide interactive ways to discuss the uses of epidemiology. These are only preliminary ideas, but I am confident that science teachers will have a better grasp of how to integrate this new discipline into their curricula.[9]

## "EARTHLY SELF-REALIZATION"

In a plea to make epidemiology accessible to senior citizens, allow me to take a very broad (but inspiring) perspective: the concept of "earthly self-realization" proposed by the late historian Richard Fogel. It may seem like a long shot, but I believe the concept is highly relevant to this chapter's topic because having access to health knowledge can help individuals "realize" their full potential, culturally and physiologically.

Fogel first invokes the growing importance of leisure time in human life. After deducting ten hours for sleep, meals, and essential hygiene, there remain fourteen hours a day to spend doing productive activities. The fraction of these fourteen hours spent working to earn a living has declined from 80 percent in 1880 to 41 percent today. Fogel predicts it will shrink further to 25 percent by 2040.[10]

His second observation is that the usage of free time has evolved. He attributes this evolution to a trend toward deemphasizing the pursuit of money and social status in favor of social life, cultural and spiritual values, and good health. Fogel cites a (now old) poll conducted in the United States showing that between 1990 and 1995 some employed adults had declined a promotion (8 percent), reduced their commitments (16 percent), lowered their material expectations (15 percent), or moved to a place because it offered a quieter lifestyle (24 percent).[11]

More free time can mean more time spent traveling, exercising, and attending music and theater performances. These amenities of life are no longer solely reserved for the rich as they were only one hundred years ago. An important component of self-realization is the continuation of education beyond job training in order to better understand ourselves and the world we live in. And here is where epidemiologic literacy naturally chimes in.

Fogel was banking on a scenario in which a typical citizen would have more than fifty hours per week of leisure time before retiring at an average age of fifty-five and an additional thirty-five years of full-time leisure thereafter.[12] Clearly, the economic trends do not coincide with such optimistic assumptions. The current economic marasmus may cast doubts about whether resources will still be available to subsidize billions of person-years of leisure activity for people living on the margins of the labor market. It is beyond my expertise to tell whether Fogel's vision is irremediable. I hope that it is not, but even if it were only a remote perspective, it does not detract from the fact that self-realization would still be, as Fogel puts it, "one of the fundamental driving forces of humanity, on a par with the most basic material needs."[13]

Health is a priority in the realization of one's self, and as Internet search trends have already shown, we can expect a demand for acquiring the basics of epidemiologic literacy in order to gain the skills needed to navigate the flow of accessible health information and better communicate with health professionals. Aside from the meeting of our personal interests, wouldn't society at large be better prepared to face acute health crises, such as epidemic threats, and to make key public-health decisions if it could count on the active involvement of citizens literate in epidemiology?

# 16

---

# BEYOND EPIDEMIOLOGY

I PLEAD guilty for two oversimplifications I made in the previous chapters. The first is that, for the sake of clarity, I equated epidemiology with the practice of group comparisons. Epidemiology is of course much more than that. History attests that epidemiologists are scientists motivated primarily by the solution of major health problems in public health and in clinical medicine. We have seen in this book that since the appearance in 1662 of the first solid root of what would become the science of epidemiology, epidemiologists were involved in discovering effective means to prevent or treat the plague, smallpox, scurvy, cholera, puerperal fever, tuberculosis, typhoid fever, many types of cancer and cardiovascular diseases, and, today, infectious, neurologic and metabolic disorders. In clinical medicine, they showed that smallpox inoculation was effective for prevention, that fevers and pneumonia did not respond to bloodletting, that streptomycin was effective against tuberculosis, and that drugs had side effects, and they provided the core of the methodology of randomized clinical trials, clinical decision analysis, and evidence-based medicine. In all these matters and many others, improving the health of populations was the motivating factor. An expertise in group comparison does not suffice to make a difference in people's health. Epidemiologists study biology, sociology, economics, history, and health policy to improve their theories. They closely track the evolution of technology to refine their measurements. The history of epidemiology has many facets.[1] The picture is not black or white. Of its fifty shades of gray, if I may say, I chose to explore the evolution of group comparisons because, in my view, epidemiologists' ability to design and perform group comparisons is what primarily distinguishes them from other scientists.

The second oversimplification of the previous chapters was the pretense that epidemiology produced objective results allowing us to neatly separate knowledge from beliefs. Things are more complicated, even considering my modest definition of health knowledge. As I said up front in the prologue, health knowledge does not mean truth but comprises the products of a type of scientific experimentation consisting in comparing groups of people. Nevertheless, epidemiology deals with human beings and society, and as human beings and citizens in society we tend to be partial toward epidemiologic results. There exist the methods but also the beliefs that animate us when we use them. It is not like the chemical formula of water, $H_2O$, on which we can get an easy consensus. No group comparison can necessarily make us all agree about the health risks of tobacco or about whether vaccines cause autism or not.

Altogether, the full picture of epidemiology is more complex than the impression of the contribution of group comparisons to health knowledge that may linger on at the end of this account. I therefore use this penultimate chapter to discuss some conceptually more difficult issues emanating from epidemiology that also belong to the humanities and social sciences, in which the distinction between belief and knowledge dwindles and sometimes become elusive.

## NORMAL AND ABNORMAL

Consider Julie, whose doctor tells her that her high blood cholesterol is abnormal. Yet Julie feels normal. She will most likely never suffer from the consequences of her high blood cholesterol level. Say that the lifetime risk of heart attack in women with a high blood cholesterol is 3 percent, Julie has a 97 percent chance of not suffering from a heart attack. However, hypercholesterolemia is a common trait among adults. A 3 percent risk is not trivial. It translates into a large excess of heart attacks. At the population level, hypercholesterolemia can therefore be viewed as abnormal because preventing it can predictably save many lives.

We think of health as being a normal state and of disease as an abnormal state. But in this example, what is the "normal" state? There is no objective answer to this question, and viewpoints have evolved during the past fifty years.

In the 1960s, it was usual to define as abnormal a characteristic that was rarely seen among young healthy adults.[2] To determine the limits of normal cholesterol, one would measure the blood cholesterol of one hundred healthy young people, draw the nearly bell-shaped distribution of the observed values, and define the 2.5 percent lowest and the 2.5 percent highest values as abnormal. Thus, abnormal values amounted to 5 percent, and the remaining 95 percent of the values were "normal." In the hospital where I trained as a medical doctor, the cut-offs separating normal and abnormal values had been derived from blood obtained from one hundred healthy nurses. When reporting a patient's laboratory results in his or her medical chart, we added a little red triangle when the blood cholesterol was lower than 125 milligrams per deciliter (3.2 millimoles per liter) or greater than 280 milligrams per deciliter (7.2 millimoles per liter). All values in between were "normal." This approach did not involve group comparisons.

But today a blood cholesterol value greater than 250 milligrams per deciliter (6.5 millimoles per liter) is considered "abnormal." What happened? Why do we have a different criterion for blood cholesterol normality now than we did only thirty years ago?

In the 1980s, a new viewpoint was adopted that integrated recent results from group comparisons. A blood cholesterol level was deemed abnormal if people exhibiting this level of blood cholesterol were at higher risk of heart attack than people with another level of blood cholesterol. Population studies indicated that the risk of heart attack was relatively constant up to total cholesterol values of 200 milligrams per deciliter, increased moderately for between 200 and 250 milligrams per deciliter, and then increased sharply for more than 250 milligrams per deciliter. The new philosophy consisted in considering that blood cholesterol values were "borderline" if they ranged between 200 and 250 milligrams per deciliter (5.2–6.2 millimoles per liter) and were "abnormal" when greater than 250 milligrams per deciliter.[3] These are now the "normal values" that you would find on your own laboratory report if you had your blood cholesterol checked recently.

Thus, Julie's doctor informs her that her blood cholesterol is abnormal because in the population her level of hypercholesterolemia is associated with a greater risk of heart attack. Julie, however, is not diseased, and her blood cholesterol level will most likely never affect her health.

The reverse situation also occurs. What looks abnormal in an individual may be normal for a population. Consider the case of spinal disc herniation. A vertebral disk is a kind of rubbery cushion between two stacked spine bones, or vertebrae. When it bulges and compresses a vertebral nerve, it can produce pain, numbness, incontinence, and loss of sensation in the thighs, back of the legs, and around the rectum. Is it not obviously abnormal to find a herniated disk or degenerative changes in the spine on a CT scan? Well, not necessarily. It depends on what your expectations are. Should the spine of a fifty-year-old man who has no complaints and feels "normal" look like the perfect spine described in anatomy books? According to doctors in Cleveland, 20 to 25 percent of people who climb into a scanner have a herniated disk, and as many as 60 percent of healthy adults with no back pain have degenerative changes in their spines.[4] What should these doctors conclude? What is the criterion for normality? The perfect spine described in medical textbooks or the typical spine observed in their patients' population of origin? What would you say?

Thanks to the large and repeated health surveys now available for an increasing number of populations, we have a growing amount of data that can show the distribution of health-related traits and risk factors in populations. We can follow their evolution across time.[5] These repeated surveys indicate what is typical in the population. They don't provide an objective criterion for separating the normal from the pathological, but they may at least inform prevention strategies. If Julie's cholesterol is high, and the majority of the other women her age in her community also exhibits high cholesterol, the problem might lie in the community's behaviors, and some form of intervention may be necessary. The culprit might be poor access to a balanced diet or insufficient physical activity because of a dearth of parks, sidewalks, or pedestrian areas in her neighborhood or because of excessive income inequality. It is necessary to improve the context in which Julie and other women of her age tend to have abnormal cholesterol levels. Julie's health can be improved on an individual basis, too, but this may be less effective than going to the root of the problem. Inversely, if John, twenty-five, has an exceptionally high blood cholesterol level for a man of his age, he may have an atypical lifestyle or some genetic susceptibility. Acting at the individual level may be effective here.

The bottom line is that population risks and their comparisons can guide the distinction between health and disease or the definition of what is normal and what is not, but they do not provide objective criteria thereof. The viewpoint of the individual does not necessarily coincide with that of the community. The location of the dividing line lies beyond epidemiology.

## INDIVIDUAL, SOCIETY, AND FREE WILL

How free are we in our interpretation of health knowledge? There are perturbing observations in populations suggesting that our ability to separate them from beliefs is modified by the characteristics of our community.

Consider the constancy of crime frequency across time in a given population. How can we explain its likeliness to remain stable from year to year? Our perception of individual crimes is that the place and time at which they occur are unpredictable. But the number of crimes that will occur in a particular community in a particular year is predictable. Why? Adolphe Quetelet, as we saw in chapter 4, gave an extreme answer: he believed that crimes were perpetrated by society behaving as a collective individual. He viewed criminals as randomly selected agents of a predetermined scenario.

Even without negating the reality of individual free will, some observations are perplexing. The demographer Sully Ledermann observed that there were more heavy drinkers in a community if that community drank on average more alcohol than another community.[6] Of course, he ruled out the fact that this was because a small group of very heavy drinkers pulled the average up. The whole population was affected, as if in the communities with more heavy drinkers, everyone tended to drink more than in communities with fewer heavy drinkers. Vice versa, in populations less inclined to drink alcohol, the proportion of heavy drinkers was smaller. This observation contradicted the common belief that each population had its immutable core of pathological alcoholics.

Ledermann died too young to explore these ideas in more depth, but the epidemiologist Geoffrey Rose generalized Ledermann's approach to

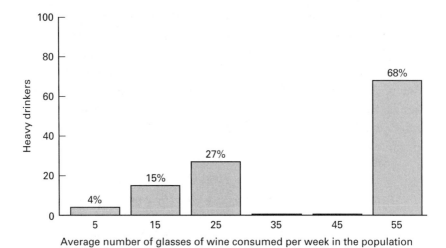

Average number of glasses of wine consumed per week in the population

FIGURE 16.1 **Proportion of Heavy Drinkers in a Population**

Relationship between mean alcohol consumption (expressed in glasses of wine consumed per week) and the proportion of those in that population who drink at least three glasses of wine per day (heavy drinkers).

*Source*: Data from the Intersalt study conducted in fifty-two populations and five continents. Adapted from Rose and Day 1990.

areas such as blood pressure, weight-to-height ratio (or body-mass index), alcohol, and salt consumption. In each of these examples, Rose confirmed Ledermann's postulate: the population mean predicted the number of deviant individuals.[7]

Figure 16.1 shows the results about alcohol consumption from the Intersalt study:[8] the proportion of heavy drinkers, defined as people drinking more than three glasses of wine per day, increases proportionally with the mean alcohol consumption in the population. The bars show that there are 4 percent of heavy drinkers in a population that drinks five glasses of wine per week on average. This proportion of heavy drinkers climbs to 15 percent for a mean consumption of fifteen glasses of wine per week— or two glasses of wine per day, corresponding to the situation in France and the United States.[9] And so on. The population at the far right of the figure consumes the equivalent of fifty-five glasses of wine per week on average. But even this unusually high figure is consistent with the general conclusion that for every additional glass of wine consumed on average, we should expect an additional one percent of heavy drinkers.

In other words, the proportion of heavy drinkers can be predicted based on the mean quantity of alcohol consumption in a population. What happened to free will? These data suggest that there cannot be a simple relation between individual decisions (to be a heavy drinker or not) and the epidemiologic knowledge about the relative health risks associated with heavy drinking (as opposed to moderate or no drinking). Our relation to knowledge (when we can access it) is likely to be modified by characteristics of the community to which we belong.[10]

## NUMBERS NEEDED

The Hippocratic Oath, which is the ethical standard among doctors worldwide, states: "I will prescribe regimens for the good of my patients according to my ability and my judgment." But what happens when the good of the individual patient does not coincide with that of the population?

Many decisions and interventions in modern medical practice and public health can benefit the community more than the individuals involved in the decision or the intervention. Group comparison provides a tool for quantifying the relative benefit for the individual versus for the community. The number needed to treat (NNT, see chapter 11) indicates how many people need to receive a medical treatment or comply with preventive or therapeutic measures in order to avoid one excess health event. For example, a risk difference of 20 percent implies that five people (100/20) need to be treated in order to avoid one health event that would have occurred had these five people not been treated.

Here are the NNTs computable in the examples given in this book:

- 730 women who exercise vigorously for five hours or more per week for one year will contribute to preventing one case of breast cancer (figure 1.1)
- For 667 people taking a daily aspirin for a year, one expected heart attack will not take place (chapter 1)
- Of five tuberculous patients treated with streptomycin, one will not die (figure 10.1)

- For 29 women using (for one year) a vaginal gel containing tenofovir, one will be spared from HIV infection (figure 11.1)
- 714 people must participate in a multirisk factor prevention program for seven years to prevent one heart attack (figure 12.1)
- 72 men need to take an antioxidant vitamin and mineral cocktail for seven years to prevent one case of cancer (figure 12.2)
- One heart attack will be prevented for every 5,000 women eliminating transfat from their diet for one year (chapter 12)
- 1,667 women ages forty to forty-nine or 556 women ages fifty to sixty-three need to be mammographically screened for seven years to prevent one death (figure 13.1)
- Among 1,429 women who take hormonal replacement therapy after menopause, one excess case of heart attack will occur per year (figure 14.1)

A treatment that less than twenty people need to take for one year to benefit at least one person is a rare thing to come by. Intuitively, it may seem that treating fewer people but focusing in those with a high risk of heart attack, breast cancer, and so on would decrease the NNT. Simple computations, as in appendix 4, show that this is not necessarily so: twice as many cases of lung cancer occur among smokers of a pack or less per day than among those who smoke more than a pack per day. Why? Because there are many more light and moderate smokers than there are heavy smokers. The risk among light and moderate smokers is smaller than that of heavy smokers, but they are more numerous. A small risk applied to a large number of people can generate more excess cases than a large risk that is applied to a small fraction of the population.

Thus, group comparisons provide a gauge, the NNT, to quantify the relative interests of the individual and the population. There is, however, no objective criterion to locate the optimal balance between these sometimes competing interests. The decision lies beyond epidemiology.

## GOODMAN'S TEST

We have now reached a delicate point in this book. I have suggested in the previous chapters that group comparisons were an apt criterion to "separate" beliefs from knowledge. The reality is that it is impossible to completely disconnect beliefs and knowledge. Our life experiences, background, scientific knowledge, and beliefs matter when interpreting the findings of a group comparison. We are not impartial regarding any study results. Our a priori expectations or biases pop up when we confront health information. This is not news. This idea has been encapsulated into a mathematical theorem that is about as old as epidemiology and group comparisons.

Around 1750, Reverend Thomas Bayes in England expressed the relation between beliefs and finds in a celebrated theorem named after him, which I will loosely summarize as follows:

New Beliefs = Prior Beliefs × Knowledge.

Our "prior beliefs" comprise all we know on a topic as well as our view of society and the world. Think of tobacco, coffee, oral contraception, vitamins, fruits and vegetables, air pollution, X-rays, and so on. Do you feel as likely to accept findings suggesting that they present some health risks as you would for findings suggesting that they are benign? I don't. Take coffee. It would cost me to be disenfranchised from my two miniature daily cups. My take on the epidemiologic evidence is that no health risk from coffee has been established. When confronted with the results of a new group comparison, I first confront it with my expectations. Afterward, I have new expectations, but unless extremely compelling evidence of risk were racked up, the comparison would not affect my current beliefs. The anecdote of the man who said he could not tell how light American coffee was, but that the American water he had for breakfast was very strong would immediately remind me how difficult it is to measure coffee intake (e.g., Should the unit be the volume, the content in caffeine, the content of methyl xanthine, the number of cups per day?) and make me relativize the finding. And I may easily find solace in reports of group comparisons suggesting that coffee drinkers live longer or at a lower risk of Alzheimer's. The latter evidence may not be stronger, but it is closer to my current belief.

Aren't you also more or less susceptible to believe new information according to what your prior beliefs are? Please consider taking Goodman's test.

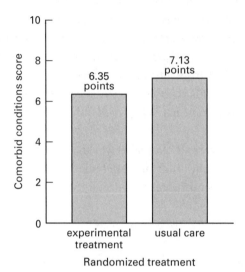

FIGURE 16.2 **Comorbid Conditions Score**
**in Coronary Care Unit, Kansas City, 1999**

Score of complications occurring after admission in a coronary care unit for a heart problem according to the random allocation to either an experimental treatment for 466 patients or usual care for 524 patients, Kansas City, in 1999. A low score means fewer complications. There is no upper limit, but a score of 10 is very high.

Professor Steven Goodman is an epidemiologist and associate dean of clinical research at Stanford University in Palo Alto, California. He devised a test based on an RCT. The trial, published in an excellent American medical journal, assessed the efficacy of a prescribed treatment—at this point, I will not disclose the type of treatment—in addition to the usual care given to reduce overall adverse events and length of stay for patients admitted to a coronary care unit. The outcome was expressed as a score on a scale of clinical complications: the lowest value, 1, corresponded to minor complications, and the scores went up as a function of more severe complications, such as the need for a pacemaker, coronary artery dilatation, cardiac arrest, or death.

Figure 16.2 shows the results of this RCT conducted among patients admitted to a coronary care unit. Half were randomly allocated to an experimental treatment in addition to the usual coronary care, and the other half received only the usual coronary care. The average score of clinical complication was 6.35 in the intervention group, which corresponded to a score reduction of 0.78 from the score in the usual care group. The intervention reduced the risk of severe complications.

What do you think? Was the experimental treatment effective? If you were admitted to a coronary care unit, would you prefer to receive the experimental treatment or just the usual care? Would it matter at all?

Mind that if you are admitted to a coronary care unit, death is looming. The fraction of a complication point prevented by the treatment can be precious. If you are concerned over whether the finding is statistically significant or not, refer to note 11.[11]

Have you decided?

Now, here is the missing piece of information: the experimental treatment was a prayer. A prayer.[12] The study consisted of randomly allocating patients to an "intercessory" prayer prayed by someone unknown to the sick and who did not know the sick person. The comparison group had no prayer.

Did the information about the nature of the treatment change your interpretation of the results? As far as I am concerned, I was previously indifferent and remain indifferent to the intercession because I cannot imagine a physical mechanism that can be scientifically examined by which a prayer that the patient does not know about at all might modify the evolution of a disease. But others whose religious beliefs are different than mine may give it more credence. Note that in the letters sent to the editor of the journal in which the paper was published, the demarcation line did not separate believers from atheists and agnostics. Instead readers raised methodological, epistemological (like mine), and theological arguments (Can we test God's will?) not to "believe" the results of this trial.[13] The authors of the paper, acknowledging the apparent positive effect of intercessory prayer on the complication risks in coronary care units, did not rule out that their results could have been due to chance alone and so suggested conducting similar RCTs with more patients. Some more recent trials have not confirmed the association.[14]

Goodman's test challenges our ability to stave off our biases when interpreting the results of an epidemiologic study. The test is extremely effective because it uses a quintessential example, combining science (the RCT) and an esoteric question regarding which opinions are divided. It is debatable whether one should even perform trials whose results cannot be interpreted. Nevertheless, the phenomenon revealed by Goodman's test is universal and applies to mundane issues. In general, we may be convinced by modest evidence when the results concur with what we already believe, but only very strong evidence can convert us to profoundly different beliefs. Try revisiting all the examples discussed in this book to assess how powerful the influence of prior beliefs is on our willingness to accept health knowledge.

# EPILOGUE

## The End of Epidemiology?

**IN 350** years, epidemiology migrated from the periphery of medicine and public health's focus to their center. Does it mean that it has reached its final destination? After all, for most of recorded history, doctors have aspired to understand and treat individual patients on the basis of individualized knowledge. However, aggregating information from individual patients, as epidemiologists do, inevitably means the loss of some distinguishing information because no two persons get sick in exactly the same way for exactly the same reasons.

We can therefore legitimately wonder whether epidemiology will no longer be needed the day doctors won't have to relinquish their patients' individual characteristics in order to group them. Is there an end to epidemiology? Fascinatingly, Claude Bernard, the great physiologist of the nineteenth century, answered this question positively. This epilogue will attempt to interpret his response in light of what we have learned.

Bernard was not an epidemiologist. He was born on July 12, 1813, to a modest family in the French wine region of Beaujolais. There he trained in clinical medicine but dedicated most of his professional life to laboratory work, mainly at the Collège de France in Paris. A brilliant experimenter, he made essential discoveries about the oxygenation of blood; the effects of opium on the sympathetic nervous system; the digestive function of the stomach; the physiologic actions of poisons, such as the muscular paralysis caused by curare; and the displacement of oxygen from hemoglobin by carbon monoxide.

But Bernard is remembered today primarily for his 1865 manifesto of modern medicine, *Introduction to the Study of Experimental Medicine*. The book described the new medicine emerging from hospitals and laboratories. At the time, French hospitals, staffed with doctors, treated large numbers of patients. Attending doctors managed populations of patients. They performed thousands of clinical examinations and hundreds of autopsies. The large number of observations began to reveal regularities. Counting the patients, their signs and symptoms, their treatments and outcomes helped to better characterize disease entities such as tuberculosis, typhoid, and typhus. Medical epidemiology naturally developed in these new Parisian hospitals.

Philippe Pinel, a leader of hospital medicine, gathered, organized, and tabulated medical data.[1] Pierre Louis, whose controversy with François Broussais I discussed in chapter 5, was the strong-minded proponent of the "numerical method": he counted and compared patients to assess whether treatment worked.[2]

In the laboratories, biologists, physiologists, microbiologists, and bacteriologists scrutinized the human body, its organs, fluids, cells, and functions. Rudolf Virchow, Louis Pasteur, Robert Koch, and Claude Bernard discovered the cell, the "germs," and the processes of body metabolism. Medicine was enriched by the new knowledge generated by these new sciences.

Doctors in hospitals and laboratories were driven by the same ambition to transform medicine into a science. They had a common adversary: the old school of clinicians who viewed medicine as an "art."

Benigno Risueño d'Amador, professor of pathology and general therapy in Montpellier, south of France, typified this outdated school of thought. On April 25, 1837, at a session of the French Royal Academy of Medicine, he argued that the role of doctor was to take care of individual patients and that, for individual patients, statistics could not replace clinical intuition. Medicine did not work like life insurance. If, on average, 10 percent of former patients died from a given surgical intervention, the physician could not predict who the next victim would be. The statistic was therefore "completely useless."[3]

Bernard disagreed and articulated a vision of medicine based on three principles: (1) medicine is not an art; (2) today's medicine needs epidemiology; and (3) tomorrow's medicine will be personalized.[4] What did he mean?

## MEDICINE IS NOT AN ART

Bernard had no sympathy for doctors who pretended that physicians should be artists rather than men (very few were women) of science. He found this idea "erroneous and essentially harmful to the development of experimental medicine."[5]

What is an artist? For Bernard, "an artist is a man who carries out a personal idea or feeling in a work of art." It is possible therefore to separate the artist from his work and use the work of art to judge the artist. But what can be the work of a medical artist? Therapeutic success? In that case, how would the physician know that a disease has not cured itself alone, despite the doctor's interference? For Bernard, "no physician's ability can be judged by the number of patients that he says he has cured; he must first of all prove scientifically that he, and not nature, was responsible for the cure."[6]

Thus, contradicting Risueño d'Amador's position, Bernard posited that physicians had no alternative than to act as scientists.

## TODAY'S MEDICINE NEEDS EPIDEMIOLOGY

To understand Bernard's opinion about epidemiology, we have to imagine him at work in his laboratory. To establish that the liver can store and secrete sugar, Bernard would repeatedly put a liver under continuous irrigation for forty minutes until it released a perfectly colorless and sugarless water. He would then store the liver at ambient temperature. If after twenty-four hours he consistently observed that the previously sugar-depleted organ had been refilled with sugar, he would conclude that the liver contains a substance from which sugar is formed.[7]

The statement is tested, universal, and definitive. In this type of experiment, repeated maneuvers must yield identical results. They beg an explanation if they don't: Was there a problem with the hypothesis or with the experiment? Bernard believed that it was a mistake to attribute differences between two experiments to chance or to simply calculate an average in order to rid oneself of the difference. He condemned the use of statistics and probabilities in physiology. To illustrate their absurdity, Bernard quipped about a physiologist who "took urine from a railroad station urinal through which people of all nations had travelled" in an attempt to assess the average characteristics of European urine.[8] This average would clearly have been meaningless.

Bernard also envisioned an individualized medicine based on knowledge as clear and indisputable as that which he established in his laboratory. "Scientific medicine" was going to elucidate how the normal organism functions, understand all the causes of dysfunction, and discover the means of correcting them. All knowledge would be tested by experiment and validated.

But Bernard was not a dreamer. He knew that momentous obstacles had to be overcome before medicine could become an individualized science. The exact bases of health and disease are complex, and their elucidation will take a very long time. Meanwhile, physicians have to take care of patients, establish diagnoses, and prescribe treatments even when they do not know exactly what causes the disease and how treatments work. Thus, medicine cannot yet entirely rely on physiology. Some of its health knowledge has to come from group comparisons. This explains why Bernard's opposition to the use of statistics in physiology did not extend to the use of statistics in medical practice evaluation.

Bernard did not use the term *epidemiology*, but he was clearly thinking of his colleagues who counted, grouped, and compared patients while practicing medicine in hospitals. It was an early form of evidence-based medicine—medicine "based on statistics which collect and *compare* cases which are analogous or more or less similar in their outer characteristics, but undefined as to their immediate cause."[9]

This evidence-based medicine had to "necessarily precede exact medicine!" Group comparisons represented an intermediary stage of medicine between old-school quacks who viewed themselves as artists and the exact scientific medicine elaborated in physiology laboratories. There seems to have been no doubt in Bernard's mind that "the *comparative experiment* [was] indispensable to scientific experimental medicine; without it a physician walks at random and becomes the plaything of endless illusions"[10]

A doctor who observes that a patient improves after being prescribed a treatment extols the treatment. Indeed, physicians often pride themselves on curing all their patients with a remedy, but, for Bernard, "the first thing to ask them is whether they tried to abstain, i.e., not treating other patients; for how can they otherwise know whether the remedy or nature cured the patients?"[11]

Thus, does the subhead "Today's Medicine Needs Epidemiology" overstate Bernard's view? The first question he asked about an alleged therapeutic knowledge was: Have you performed a "comparative experiment" or, in modern terms, a group comparison? In the controversy about the efficacy of bloodletting for treating pneumonia, Bernard was clearly on the side of the "numerical method" involving the comparison of the average mortality of patients bled earlier versus those bled later: "We may be subject daily to the greatest illusions about the value of treatment if we do not have recourse to comparative experiment. I shall recall only one recent example concerning the treatment of pneumonia. A comparative experiment showed, in fact, that treatment of pneumonia by bleeding, which was believed most efficacious, is a mere therapeutic illusion."[12] Bernard, referring to Louis's study (described in chapter 5), rejected bloodletting more radically than Louis, who did not rule out that bleeding could be used beneficially in some situations.

Bernard was a visionary. He understood that group comparisons would continue to contribute to medical knowledge. Medical and public-health students are taught today that epidemiology, biology, and physiology are complementary disciplines. The results of group comparisons gain credibility when their results are compatible with known biologic or physiologic mechanisms. And vice versa: assessing the potential impact of biologic and physiologic observations on human health requires group comparisons.

## WILL TOMORROW'S MEDICINE BE PERSONALIZED?

What should we think of Bernard's third tenet that medicine will one day rely only upon laboratory knowledge? Does this imply that we will have identified all the mechanisms of individual illnesses and be able to cure them all? Was he a nineteenth-century utopian without any perception of a boundary in the development of the exact sciences, which had begun to overthrow a millennia of abstract, intuitive, and speculative thinking?

In Bernard's vision, medicine was bound to become a science strictly based on experimental evidence and therefore on the exact knowledge of the physiological mechanisms underlying a disease process or the effect of a treatment. Take Bernard's example of the itch: "[F]ormerly, we knew the itch only empirically. Then we guessed about lesions in the itch and collected statistics on the value of one salve or another for curing the disease. Now that the cause of the itch is known and experimentally determined, it has all become scientific and empiricism has disappeared. . . . [W]e cure it always without exception."[13]

"We cure it always without exception": that is the Holy Grail! Once the cause of a disease is known, there is no need for probabilities anymore. Medicine becomes an exact science. It does not need to rely on the approximate knowledge derived from group comparisons.[14] The day physicians have an effective, personalized solution for each patient, they can ditch epidemiology.

Something is eminently correct in Bernard's view. His vision of scientific medicine can fully meet our expectations as individuals. Our quest for knowledge will not be put to rest before the exact mechanisms underlying health and disease are fully discovered. This is the only form of knowledge that can stand completely on its own. We wish ultimately for individual certainty in place of epidemiologic methods that can provide only population-derived probabilities.

Epidemiology identifies the causes of health and disease in populations, but each of us is seeking health knowledge that is individualized. In our inner self, we have not abandoned the ambition of ancient holistic medicines to fully understand the determinants of each individual's health.

Fully personalized human medicine is, however, a mirage. Chance puts it out of reach of the human mind. Each individual will always be unique. Individual response to treatment will always escape exact prediction. But does that matter? This ideal goal has always been what we strive for, and we will never abandon it. It is the motivation behind medical research. It is also a useful mirage. Let's reach it! Until we do, let's not forget that group comparisons remain the indispensable source of knowledge for prevention and therapy—or, as Bernard would have put it, our only protection against endless illusions.

Thus, "no end in sight" can be the answer to this chapter's title and the conclusion of this historical primer on how society embraced epidemiology as a science to solve enigmas of health and disease. We have backtracked the path taken by epidemiology to come to the center of knowledge acquisition in medicine and public health. Beginning with the plague, group comparisons have systematically been used to unravel scientific mysteries underlying the major health challenges of the time. Epidemiology plays a considerable role in our every day life. Why are we waiting to add its two essential concepts, group comparisons and population thinking, to the school curricula?

# APPENDIX 1

## INTERACTION OF CAUSES

IN ITS most extreme case, when two causes interact, they have no effect other than a joint effect. Consider the case of favism.

Ingestion of the large and flat fava beans can lead to severe anemia among people whose red blood cells lack an enzyme called glucose-6-phosphate dehydrogenase (G6PD). However, ingestion of fava beans in the absence of the G6PD deficiency does not cause anemia, nor does anemia occur in the G6PD deficient person in the absence of fava bean consumption. Fava beans and G6PD deficiency produce anemia jointly. There is thus interaction between fava bean ingestion and G6PD deficiency with respect to the risk of anemia.

The principle of interaction is used when simultaneously prescribing several drugs (multitherapy) aimed at killing bacteria or viruses that are resistant to each of these drugs in isolation (monotherapy), but sensitive to these same drugs when prescribed jointly.

More generally, two causes interact when their individual effects do not simply add up. Take the case of no interaction first: if cause A alone increases the risk by 10 percent and cause B alone increases the risk by 5 percent, A and B jointly increase the risk by 15 percent (10 percent + 5 percent). In contrast, when A and B interact, their joint effect will be either smaller than 15 percent if A and B are antagonistic or greater than 15 percent if A and B act synergistically.

Excess risk of A without B = 10%.
Excess risk of B without A = 5%.
Joint excess risk of A and B without interaction = 10% + 5% = 15%.

Joint excess risk of A and B if they interact: different (smaller or greater) than 15%.

Let us apply this principle to our example in chapter 2. Suppose that another group comparison shows that ulcers are more common in the spring season than during the rest of the year. This evidence is in addition to the evidence regarding the effect of stress on the risk of duodenal ulcer. What happens when we are stressed and it is spring? How can we measure the joint effect of stress and season? If we assume no interaction, we can simply add the stress effect and the spring effect to get the answer. This is the reductionist approach. By contrast, in the holistic approach the joint occurrence of stress and spring creates a new condition distinct from that resulting from stress alone or from spring alone. The new condition requires a particular management. The joint effect of two causes, stress and season, is not assumed as a simple combination of their individual effects. Stress and season "interact."

In holistic thinking, all causes interact, and each additional cause creates a new diagnosis susceptible to a different therapy. Because holistic explanatory models are saturated with interactions, it is not possible in the current state of our analytic techniques to test their validity.

# APPENDIX 2

## ODDS RATIO AND RISK RATIO

WE WILL compute the Cornfield odds ratio from the results of the case–control study conducted by Richard Doll and A. Bradford Hill (1950). There were 99.7 percent tobacco smokers among the cases and 95.8 percent among the controls.

We first divide each of these proportions of smokers by the complementary proportions of nonsmokers:

99.7/0.3 = 332, and 95.8/4.2 = 22.8.

Such ratios are called "odds," like those used in horse betting. A horse has an odds of four to one if it has an 80 percent chance of losing the race and a 20 percent chance of winning it (80 percent versus 20 percent = 4 versus 1). In the case–control study, the odds of being a smoker were 99.7 percent (of losing against smoking, if I might put it this way) versus 0.3 percent among the lung cancer cases. Among the controls, the odds were 95.8 percent versus 4.2 percent.

Second, we divide the odds among the *cases* by the odds among the *controls* to get the odds ratio:

Odds ratio = (99.7/0.3)/(95.8/4.2) =14.6.

This odds ratio means that cases were 14.6 times more likely to smoke than the controls.

Third, we compare this odds ratio with the risk ratio obtained by Doll and Hill when they extrapolated the results from the controls to the whole population of Great London:

Risk ratio = 17 per 100,000/1.2 per 100,000 = 14.2.

This risk ratio means that smokers were 14.2 times more likely to get lung cancer than nonsmokers.

The odds ratio of 14.6 is a little bit higher than the risk ratio of 14.2. Odds ratios are always more extreme than risk ratios. But the important point is that they have (approximately) the same magnitude: 14 times. They can therefore be interpreted in the same way.

The case–control study provides the odds ratio, but its value is usually similar to the risk ratio. It is therefore unnecessary to know whether the 14 came from a ratio of odds or a ratio of risks. We can say, in both situations, that smokers had fourteen times greater risk of developing lung cancer than nonsmokers.

Thanks to Bayes Theorem, the proportions of smokers, 99.7 percent and 95.8 percent, have been transformed into an odds ratio of 14, which can also be interpreted as a risk ratio of 14.

# APPENDIX 3

## WHY COHORT AND CASE–CONTROL STUDIES CONCUR

AS EXPLAINED in chapter 7, a *cohort* study consists of comparing the occurrence of disease between exposed and nonexposed people, whereas the *case–control* study compares the past exposure of patients with the disease and that of people without. Did you notice that the two studies of smoking and lung cancer conducted by Richard Doll and A. Bradford Hill (1950, 1964) also discussed in chapter 7, which were evidently different in their design—the 1950 case–control study compared a group of cases of lung cancer with a control group free of lung cancer, and the 1964 cohort study conducted a follow-up of smokers and nonsmokers over ten years—yielded an identical result: people who ever smoked were fourteen times more likely to develop lung cancer than never smokers?

This precise identity of the result was to some extent due to chance, but the overall similarity is not chance at all. It is actually expected that a cohort study and a case–control study performed among similar populations yield the same result. Understanding this expectation is crucial for interpreting the results of case–control studies when they are reported in a newspaper article. You may have noticed that newspaper articles will say, for example, that cell phone users have a higher "risk" of developing some form of brain cancer, even though the study consisted in comparing patients having developed brain cancer with controls without brain cancer and no risk was computed. In this appendix, I explain why this interpretation of a case–control study is perfectly legitimate.

There is no magic, but there is a trick. Understanding how the trick works requires a small twist of the imagination. Instead of thinking of the case–control study as the results of selecting cases and controls and comparing them on past exposure, we should reflect on the underlying phenomenon: the origin of the cases and controls. As life goes on, patients arise out of exposed and unexposed populations. To perform a case–control study, we pick these patients as they occur over time and treat them as "cases." Each time a case is ascertained, we also pick as controls comparable people who are free of disease in the same populations.

Let's first focus on the exposed and unexposed populations. Consider the simple scenario of a perfectly imaginary cohort with four subjects. First, a male smoker is followed across time, and he develops lung cancer after one year of follow-up. The control for that patient is a person who is alive and free of lung cancer at the time the case is diagnosed. The investigators in the study will ascertain whether the control ever smoked. A second male, a nonsmoker, develops lung cancer after four years of follow-up; he too will be matched with a person, a control, who has not developed lung cancer during the first four years. This second control is also selected independently of whether he smokes or not. The interviews of the two controls reveal that the first smokes and the second does not. At the end of the study, the data are analyzed. Among the patients, one smokes, and the other does not. Among the controls, one smokes, and the other does not. There seems to be no difference; however, that is a wrong conclusion. This conclusion would ignore the fact that the two pairs are not identical. In the first pair, the patient developed the disease after one year, and in the second pair the patient developed the disease after four years. The time of occurrence of lung cancer is important information.

We can take this time information into account in the analysis if we consider that each control represents a certain amount of person-time free of disease. In our first pair, the control is someone who remained free of lung cancer for at least one year—that is, one person-year. In the second pair, the control is someone who remained free of lung cancer for at least four years—that is, four person-years. Thus, the comparison of the two pairs would be fairer if the first were viewed as one patient and one person-year and the second as one patient and four person-years. From an exposure perspective, there is one lung cancer patient for one person-year among smokers and one lung cancer patient for four person-years among the nonsmokers. This new perspective leads to the correct conclusion. Among smokers, there is one case per year; among nonsmokers, there is one case every four years, or

0.25 cases per year. The rate ratio is 4 (1/0.25): lung cancer occurs four times more quickly among smokers than among nonsmokers.[1] Let's see how this can be related to deriving rate ratios from a case–control study.

Consider the 649 case–control pairs in the London tobacco and lung cancer study in chapter 7. A total of 647 of the cases smoked, and 2 did not. The cases occurred over two years of follow-up. If we knew the total number of person-times accrued by the controls, we could compute rates of lung cancer. A rate is calculated by dividing the number of cases by person-times, as we did in the imaginary cohort example of two pairs. We could do this for the smokers and the nonsmokers. The number of smoking cases divided by the number of smoking person-times would be the rate of lung cancer among smokers. The number of nonsmoking cases divided by the number of nonsmoking person-times would be the rate of lung cancer among nonsmokers. Unfortunately, none of these person-times can be measured in a case–control study.

However, and here is where the small twist of the imagination comes in, the *ratio* of smoking person-years over nonsmoking person-years can be derived from a case–control study.

Because smoking causes lung cancer, people who survive long enough to still be eligible as controls after one, two, three, or more years are increasingly more likely to be nonsmokers. This change of distribution of smoking habits in controls over time will be reflected in the ratio of smoking over nonsmoking controls. Actually, in the lung cancer case–control study, the ratio of smoking controls over nonsmoking controls is identical to the ratio of smoking person-years over nonsmoking person-years that would be measured in a cohort study.

This is very useful. The link between cohort and case–control studies can be now shown in three simple steps. We start with the rate ratio that could be computed in a cohort study:

Rate ratio of lung cancer = [Smoking cases (A) over smoking person-times (B)] ÷ [nonsmoking cases (C) over nonsmoking person-times (D)].

In other words,

Rate ratio = A/B ÷ C/D.

The second step consists in reorganizing the equation: A/B ÷ C/D is equivalent to A/C ÷ B/D.

Rate ratio = [Smoking cases over nonsmoking cases] ÷ [smoking person-times over nonsmoking person-times].

Third, here comes the small twist again, the value of the ratio [smoking person-times over nonsmoking person-times] is identical to the ratio of [smoking controls over nonsmoking controls]. We can therefore substitute one ratio by the other:

Rate ratio = [smoking cases over nonsmoking cases] ÷ [smoking controls over nonsmoking controls].

Let's calculate the latter expression of the rate ratio from the London 1950 tobacco–lung cancer case–control study:

Rate ratio of lung cancer = 647/2 ÷ 622/27 = 14.

We get the same rate ratio if we replace the numbers of cases and controls by the exact proportions of smokers and nonsmokers:

Rate ratio of lung cancer = 99.69/0.31 ÷ 95.84/4.16 = 14.

This is the only magic Doll and Hill used to transform the proportion of smokers among the cases, 99.7 percent, and the proportion of smokers among the controls, 95.8 percent, into a rate ratio of 14.[2] This is also the reason why a newspaper article summarizing the results of a case–control study will not report the proportions of exposure, but the rate ratio instead.

Introductory courses of epidemiology still teach that the rate ratio is only approximated by the odds ratio computed in a case–control study, as described in appendix 2. The arithmetical explanation appears easier to grasp than the conceptual explanation given here. However, as a rule, case–control studies directly provide rate ratios.[3]

# APPENDIX 4

## WHERE DO THE CASES OF LUNG CANCER COME FROM?

TO ILLUSTRATE why most cases of lung cancer occur in moderate smokers, I am approximating data from 2011 in the United States, but the same demonstration could be made for most, and probably all, populations.

Consider that there are in the United States 60 million moderate smokers who smoke a pack of cigarettes a day or less. They represent 20 percent of the total US population. There is another 3 percent of the population, or 9 million, who are heavy smokers of more than a pack of cigarettes per day. Let us assume that the annual risk of lung cancer is 3 per 1,000 for the moderate smokers and 10 per 1,000 for the heavy smokers.

Thus, 20 percent of the population has an annual risk of 1 per 1,000, and 3 percent of the population has an annual risk of 10 per 1,000. The expected number of cases of lung cancer can be computed as follows:

3/1,000/year × 60 million = 180,000 cases per year among the moderate
 smokers.
10/1,000/year × 9 million = 90,000 cases per year among the heavy
 smokers.

Therefore, almost twice as many cases of lung cancer would be expected to occur among moderate smokers (180,000 cases) than among heavy smokers (90,000 cases).

# NOTES

## PREFACE TO THE ENGLISH EDITION

1. Morabia 2004a.


## PROLOGUE: A SCIENCE NAMED EPIDEMIOLOGY

1. Pettenkofer 1941, 42.
2. Quoted in Leonhardt 2009.
3. Hope 2010.
4. Walsh 2010.
5. Kirkey 2011.
6. The *ABC News* website has a section on epidemiology, http://abcnews.go.com/topics/news/healthcare/epidemiology.htm, as does *Fox News*, http://www.foxnews.com/topics/healthcare/epidemiology.htm.
7. For an elaboration on the origin of the terms *epidemiology* and *epidemiologist*, see Martin and Martin-Granel 2006.
8. Morabia et al. 1996. This study was performed using the Bus Santé, a local program similar to the National Health and Nutrition Survey in the United States; see Morabia 2005.
9. Brody 1996.
10. See "Medicine and Health: Epidemiology" n.d.


## 1. COMPARING GROUPS AND THE FIFTH DIMENSION

1. Manson 2010.
2. Tehard et al. 2006.

3. In the epidemiologic jargon, a risk per unit of time is called an "incidence rate." For example, an annual risk of 38.1 per 10,000 women would be called an incidence rate of 38.1 per 10,000 per year. To stick with a minimal number of technical words, I prefer to use the word *risk* and specify whether it is annual or over a different period of time.

4. It is not always accurate to compute a thirty-year risk by multiplying the average annual risk by 30. But for breast cancer, which is a relatively rare disease, the error is small.

5. McAlonan 2008.

6. The adjective *salicylic* comes from the Latin *salix*, which means "willow tree."

7. Quoted in Volmink 2008, 322. The effect of salicilin was rediscovered in the eighteenth century by the English reverend Edward Stone; see Stone 1764.

8. Boston Collaborative Drug Surveillance Group 1974.

9. Sanmuganathan et al. 2001.

10. $10,000/15 = x/1, x = 10,000/15 = 667$.

11. Centers for Disease Control and Prevention 2010b.

12. Centers for Disease Control and Prevention 2011.

13. Jefferson, Di, Al-Ansary, et al. 2010; Jefferson, Di, Rivetti, et al. 2010; Thomas, Jefferson, and Lasserson 2010.

14. The analysis of 23 million people vaccinated during the 2009 pandemic identified 1.6 excess cases of Guillain-Barré syndrome per million people vaccinated. These cases may have occurred by chance. See Poland, Poland, and Howe 2013; Salmon et al. 2013.

15. Centers for Disease Control and Prevention 2010a.

16. Council of Europe Parliamentary Assembly 2010, 9; see also Jefferson 2010.


## 2. PEOPLE, BUGS, AND EPIDEMICS

1. About the importance of infectious diseases in prehistoric foraging societies, see Fenner 1970; Cohen and Armalagos 1984; and Kelly 1995.

2. The vulnerability of contemporary foraging societies to modern infectious agents is described in Hill and Hurtado 1996 for the Ache of Paraguay, in Truswell and Hansen 1976 for the Bushmen !Kung of South Africa, and in Bailey 1991 for the Efe Pygmies of Northeast Africa.

3. About the evolution of the first epidemics of infectious diseases in agrarian societies, see McNeill 1977; Diamond 1999; and Wolfe, Dunavan, and Diamond 2007.

4. McNeill 1977.

5. Life in Mesoamerica before the Spanish Conquest is described in two beautiful books: Soustelle 1955 and Mann 2006.

6. Within the great trends of world epidemics, one can distinguish the history of particular epidemics. Leprosy, common during the first thousand years of our era, had practically disappeared by the nineteenth century; it probably subsided due to the rise of tuberculosis (see Donoghue et al. 2005). The Atlantic slave trade may have brought malaria and yellow fever to the Americas. However, syphilis was probably endemic in the Americas until it traveled from west to east, carried by soldiers coming back to Europe, where it first appeared at the end of the fifteenth century. Typhus devastated Europe between 1500 and 1900. A very rich bibliography includes for the plague, Gottfried 1983 and Benedictow 2006; for typhus, Zinsser 1935; for smallpox, Hopkins 2002; and for syphilis, Harper et al. 2008.

7. Sigerist 1951, 29–37.

8. A full analysis of the Chinese epidemic catalog is in Morabia 2009a. In his masterpiece *Imperial China* (1999), Frederick Mote describes the historical context and many demographical aspects of the Chinese Empire since the tenth century, but he includes very little about health and medicine. I have also used the demographic studies by Durand 1960.

9. The Chinese mode of enumeration of the population is ordinarily referred to as "censuses," but in reality they were not always periodic counts of all the inhabitants of the empire territory. The Jing dynasty (1115–1234) performed triennial enumeration, but for the Southern Song (1127–1279), the Ming (1368–1644), the Qing (1644–1911), and probably earlier dynasties, population was enumerated in permanent registers. It was hard to maintain accurate population registries over long periods of time characterized by dynastic successions, wars, invasions, and profound changes in country leadership. Moreover, not all dynasties defined a countable person the same way. People could be omitted because they did not pay taxes, were not Chinese, or were women. Some people had reasons to conceal their existence—usually to escape taxation or military service or labor draft.

10. The first trough, grossly between 1200 and 1400, corresponds to the Mongol domination by the Yuan dynasty (1272–1378), and the second, between 1650 and 1750, is the first period of the Manchu Qing dynasty (1644–1734). Major population losses may have occurred following the Mongol and Manchu conquests due to warfare and subsequent destruction of the economy, but not necessarily due to epidemic diseases. This hypothesis is consistent with the analysis of another imperial database showing that the number of rebellions and wars also peaked in the fourteenth century and the seventeenth century . Administrative failures to record populations during troubled times may have exaggerated the apparent losses.

11. McNeill 1977.

12. The term *epidemic* comes from the Greek compound of the preposition *epi*, meaning "upon," and the word *demos*, meaning "population." According to Paul Martin and Estelle Martin-Granel (2006), the term *epidemic* had different meanings in Greek

antiquity. Since the eighteenth century, it has meant recurrent attacks of the same disease.

13. What we know of the devastating epidemics before the eighteenth century was often recorded by historians and writers, not by doctors. The Greek historian Thucydides described the Plague of Athens in 430 BCE. The Byzantine historian Procopius described the Justinian Plague of 541 CE. The Italian writer Giovanni Boccaccio described life during the Black Death of the fourteenth century. Daniel Defoe wrote a novel about life in London during one of the last outbreaks of plague of the seventeenth century. In contrast, doctors made clinical observations, distinguishing bubonic from pneumonic plague, proposing holistic treatments, and speculating about the astrological causes of a disease (the Black Death was allegedly caused when Jupiter aligned with Mars and Saturn was in the fortieth degree of Aquarius).

14. "In Galen's medicine, prophylaxis and treatment were directed largely to the creation and maintenance of the proper humoral balance in each individual, *which varied from person to person* and which it took the good physician some time to know in full" (Nutton 1983, 16, emphasis added).

15. Jouanna 2001.

16. Analogies between ancient holistic medicine in China and Europe are discussed in Needham 1981.

17. Quoted in R. Porter 1997, 151.

18. Quoted in ibid., 216.

19. McNeill 1977; Diamond 1999.

20. Mann 2006.

21. De Montellano 1990.

22. Hopkins 2002.

23. Morabia 2009a.

24. "Never to accept anything for true which I did not know from evidence to be such" (Descartes 1953, 137, my translation). See the fifth and sixth sections of the *Discourse*.

25. "The second, to divide each of the difficulties under examination into as many parts as possible, and as might be necessary for its adequate solution" (Descartes 1953, 138, my translation).

26. Descartes closely followed the birth of the theory of probabilities and was well versed in the work of Blaise Pascal.

27. The main cause of duodenal ulcer is a bacterium, *Helicobacter pylori*, the absence of which in some of the cases of duodenal ulcer suggests that it may not be the unique cause. Stress might be an independent cause of this disease.

28. The study (Anda et al. 1992) consisted in enumerating all the new cases of duodenal ulcer that occurred between 1971 and 1984 among the participants of the US National Health and Nutrition Examination Survey. The 4,511 participants had not had duodenal ulcer before 1971.

29. These pioneers include James Jurin, John Artbuthnot, Thomas Nettleton, and Zabdiel Boylston. See Rusnock 2002 and Boylston 2012.

30. Boylston 2012, 212.

31. "Conduct my thoughts in such order that, by commencing with objects the simplest and easiest to know, I might ascend by little and little, and, as it were, step by step, to the knowledge of the more complex" (Descartes 1953, 138, my translation).

## 3. PLAGUE'S SHARK TEETH AND SEAMEN'S ENIGMATIC EXHAUSTION

1. The Latin title of Bacon's book is *Historia vitae et mortis*, usually translated as *History of Life and Death*. Both are easily available on line. The problem is that some of the available translations from Latin do not serve well the elegant, original Latin version, beginning with the title. A more appropriate translation would be *Accounts of Life and Death*.

2. Donaldson 2013.

3. Rosen 1958, iii.

4. Graunt [1662] 2004.

5. Morabia 2013a.

6. There were more than a one hundred plague deaths per year from 1604 to 1611, in 1625 and 1626, in 1630 and 1631, and from 1636 to 1648.

7. Graunt [1662] 2004, 36.

8. See Biraben 1975; Appleby 1980; Slack 1981.

9. Quoted in Bown 2003, 38.

10. Lind 1753. Lind's group comparison study is described and discussed in Carpenter 1986 and Troehler 2008.

11. Carpenter 1986 explains the chemistry principles that structured the medical theories of the eighteenth century.

12. According to Ulrich Troehler (2000), citrus fruits had also been proposed as a treatment by an English doctor in 1747.

13. Lind 1753.

14. Bown 2003. At Trafalgar, the English were both physically and militarily stronger.

## 4. THE MYSTERY OF THE BLUE DEATH

1. Quetelet 1869.

2. R. Porter 1997; D. Porter 1999.

3. Frank 1788.

4. Frank 1790. Frank writes: "Hoc unicum vero, uberrimam scilicet morborum originem, extremam populorum miseriam, dissipare, vel tolerabiliorem reddere

praetervideant, & vix conspicua erunt Legum sanitati publicae invigilantium beneficia" (308), which means, grossly, that the benefits of "public-health" (*sanitati publicae*) legislation will remain inconspicuous if one does not reduce or make more tolerable the main source of disease: people's extreme misery.

5. For example, Edwin Chadwick in England or Lemuel Shattuck in America. See Hamlin 1985.

6. Ibid.

7. Quoted in Barry 2005, 50.

8. Snow 1855.

9. Snow 1849, 46–47.

10. According to Jan P. Vandenbroucke, Harm Eelkman Rooda, and Marieke Beukers (1991), John Snow's work acquired its current notoriety when Wade Hampton Frost, the first American professor of epidemiology, republished in 1935 the 1855 edition of Snow's *On the Mode of Communication*.

11. Pettenkofer published in German, abundantly. Two of his essays, translated into English by Henry Sigerist, remain a captivating reading. See Sigerist 1941.

12. Mill 1882, 371.

13. Morabia 2007. The episode has been magisterially told in Evans 2005.

14. Wildner and Hofman 2008.

15. Morabia 2008b.

16. Gaffky succeeded Koch as head of the Imperial Health Office (Kaiserliches Gesundheitsamt) and then in 1905 of the Institute for Infectious Diseases (Institut fuer Infektionskrankheiten).

## 5. THE NUMERICAL METHOD

1. Bartley 1832.

2. For these portraits, go to http://www.flickr.com/photos/maulleigh/2334438721/in/set-72157604123333638.

3. It is easy today to ridicule Broussais for the leeches and the literary logorrhea, but he was a courageous man. Broussais had been surgeon on the corsair boat *Le Boungainville* and doctor of the Napoleonic army during the German campaigns. In his books, descriptions abound of sick soldiers whom he treated under difficult conditions. When France faced the threat of the cholera pandemic in 1829, the Royal Academy of Medicine asked Broussais to prepare a report, which was published in 1831 as *Rapport à l'Académie royale de médecine sur le choléra-morbus*. Broussais was highly respected by his contemporaries.

4. Ackerknecht 1986, 84.

5. "Throughout Europe, hundreds of millions of leeches were used by physicians" (Carter and Carter 2005, 7).

6. Ackerknecht 1967, 74.

7. Louis 1825.

8. Louis 1841.

9. Some modern Swiss pneumologists unanimously voted that Louis's clinical definition of the disease that affected the patients in his sample fit pneumococcal bronchopneumonia (Morabia and Rochat 2001).

10. Louis 1836, 55. Louis published his initial observations (on seventy-seven patients treated at La Charité) in 1828 (Louis 1828). In 1835, he reprinted this analysis in a book, along with new data based on twenty-nine additional pneumonia patients from La Pitié (Louis 1835). The latter text was then translated into English the following year (Louis 1836). I have previously discussed Louis's work and contribution in Morabia 1996b, 2004b, and 2009b.

11. A reanalysis of Louis's data with modern statistical methods confirms his results. See Morabia 1996b.

12. Louis did not say that bloodletting was useless. He thought it was less useful than generally believed and should be restricted to severe cases of pneumonia: "Bloodletting, notwithstanding its influence as limited, should not be neglected in inflammations which are severe and are seated in important organs" (1836, 23). He also believed that venous bloodletting was more "useful" than local bleeding and that therefore the lancet seemed to be superior to leeches. Louis's comparison suffered, however, from a main limitation: he could not guarantee that the patients bled early and those bled later were really comparable, in particular with respect to the severity of the disease. A deleterious effect of early bleeding could also have been observed if those bled earlier had more severe forms of pneumonia than those bled later. Imagine someone with a severe case of pneumonia brought to the hospital in a semicomatose state immediately after the onset of disease and then immediately bled copiously. This patient could not be compared to a patient with a less severe case of pneumonia who stays home during the acute phase but then goes to the hospital because after four days he still does not feel well and is then bled under safer conditions. If these two extreme examples were representative of the early-bled and late-bled groups, the deleterious effect of early bleeding could be explained by differences in severity of disease rather than by the timing of venosection. Louis explicitly defended his results by saying that the two groups were comparable in terms of clinical severity. See Louis 1835, 13–14.

13. On the English quantitativist doctors of the eighteenth century, see Troehler 2000. William Black's *Arithmetickal and Medical Analysis of the Diseases and Mortality of the Human Species*, published in 1789, was a nonconformist treatise that promised professional salvation to the doctors who read it: "However it may be slighted as an heretical innovation, I would strenuously recommend *Medical Arithmetick* as a guide and compass through the labyrinth of therapeutick" (117).

14. Louis was not trained in mathematics or in probability theory. He does not seem to have studied the work of statisticians, in particular that of Pierre-Simon Laplace. Also, like the British medical quantitativists of the eighteenth century, he was relatively marginal to the academic establishment. As Ulrich Troehler notes, this marginal practice gave more freedom to ambitious young doctors to be innovative and to distinguish themselves from the rest of provincial doctors (2000, 117–120).

15. For a genealogy of Louis's disciples in England and America, see Lilienfeld and Lilienfeld 1980. During his lifetime, Louis was well known in France, the United Kingdom, and the United States. He was physician to the Hôtel-Dieu; perpetual president of the Medical Society of Observation; member of the Royal Academy of Medicine and the Provincial Medical and Surgical Association of England; honorary member of the Medical Society of Massachusetts and the Medical Society of Edinburgh; and fellow of the College of Physicians, the Medical Society of Philadelphia, the Royal Academy of St. Petersburg, the Medical Society of Heidelberg, the Medical Society of Bruges, and the Medical Society of Observation of Boston.

16. Beginning at four o'clock on Sunday afternoons, new arrivals were assigned midwives. After twenty-four hours, beginning at four o'clock on Monday afternoon, new women were placed in the medical clinic. From Friday at 4:00 PM to Sunday at 4:00 PM, all new deliveries were performed by doctors. See Carter 1983.

17. Ibid.

18. Noakes et al. 2008.

19. The link with the overmortality is speculative. We cannot rule out that women also wanted to avoid being examined and delivered by men.

20. Carter and Carter 2005, 32.

## 6. EUGENICS, OYSTERS, SOUR SKIN, AND BREAST CANCER

1. Morabia, Rubenstein, and Victora 2013.

2. Refer to Fairchild and Oppenheimer 1998 on the debate regarding the efficacy of isolating patients to control tuberculosis. On the Movement for Racial Hygiene, see R. Proctor 1988 and Weindling 1989.

3. Weinberg is known today mostly for having independently discovered, with Britain's leading mathematician Godfrey Harold Hardy, a law of population genetics later known as the Hardy–Weinberg formula. See Crow 1999.

4. The original publication is Weinberg 1913. It is reanalyzed and discussed in Morabia and Guthold 2007. An English summary is available in "William Weinberg" 2009.

5. Weinberg also observed that children of the tuberculous had shorter lives if they were younger siblings, had many siblings, had parents who died at a younger age, or were of lower social class. All these associations indicated that social factors played a

more decisive role than constitutional ones. For example, consider two brothers who shared half of their genetic constitution. There is no reason to expect the younger one to have the shorter life. However, food and parents' care must have been sparser the higher a child was in the sibling count.

6. Weinberg 1913, 157. This is the first time that Weinberg mentions racial hygiene in the book.

7. Crow 1999.

8. Because all the events Weinberg studied had already occurred when he started the study, it can be specified that his study was a "retrospective" or, using a term that I prefer, "historical" cohort study.

9. Bulstrode 1902.

10. Hardy 2003a.

11. Bulstrode 1902, 130.

12. Some mysteries remain. How did Bulstrode collect data on the two people who died from enteric fever before he started his inquiry? Perhaps he interrogated their dinner companions. In particular, how was oyster consumption in the information available on the dead waiter's diet?

13. Morabia and Hardy 2005. This is what epidemiologists did in Germany to investigate the origin of the July 2011 *Escherichia coli*, which killed about twenty people and infected many thousands. See Buchholz et al. 2011.

14. Hardy 2003b.

15. Siler, Garrison, and MacNeal 1914.

16. Terris 1964, 10.

17. A 1914 editorial in the *Journal of the American Medical Association* already opposed the infectious theory and Golberger's dietary hypothesis ("The Etiology of Pellagra" 1914).

18. Goldberger, Waring, and Willets 1915, 3125. See also Goldberger, Waring, and Tanner 1923 and Morabia 2008a.

19. The results were reported in several papers published in 1920. I focus here on one of them: Goldberger, Wheeler, and Sydenstricker 1920.

20. Goldberger and Sydenstricker used an original method to assess household incomes. The mills' payroll records provided information about 90 percent of the family income, and statements by the housewife or other family members the other 10 percent. The incomes were averaged over the number of persons in the household. To allow for differences in household compositions, women's needs were counted as representing 80 percent and children's needs 50 percent of an adult man's needs. Thus, a couple and two young children would count as $1 + 0.8 + 0.5 + 0.5 = 2.8$ adult male units. Goldberger and Sydenstricker made these measures twice, in April and June, before the period during which they expected to see a rapid growth in the number of pellagra cases.

21. Marks 2003, 47; see also Roe 1973, 105, and Kraut 2003.

22. Kraut 2003.
23. Bollet 1992.
24. Carpenter 2004.
25. Lane-Claypon 1926, v.
26. Ibid., 55.
27. Press and Pharoah 2010.
28. Winkelstein 2004; Morabia 2010.

## 7. TOBACCO AND HEALTH: THE GREAT CONTROVERSY

1. Three excellent and complementary references on the history of cigarettes: Kluger 1997, Brandt 2007, and Proctor 2012.
2. Miura, Daynard, and Samet 2006.
3. Ingalls 1936, 312.
4. Roffo 1931; Proctor 2006.
5. Pearl 1938. Half a century later, in the analysis of the forty-year follow-up of the British Doctors Study, the median difference in life expectancy was also ten years, as in Pearl's 1938 study.
6. Ochsner and DeBakey 1939, 435.
7. Hoffman 1931, 67.
8. These studies are Mueller 1939 and Schairer and Schoeniger 1943; see also Schairer and Schoeniger 2001. I have published technical analyses of the two studies (Morabia 2012, 2013b).
9. See, for example, Ramsey 1925; Lane-Claypon 1926; Johnson 1929; Stocks and Karn 1933; English, Willius, and Berkson 1940.
10. "The Increase in Cancer of the Lung" 1932, 1207.
11. Quoted in "Continuing Fight" 1949.
12. "Cancer of the Lung" 1942.
13. "Cancer of the Lung" 1952.
14. Levin, Goldstein, and Gerhardt 1950.
15. Ibid., 338.
16. Wynder and Graham 1950, 336.
17. Keating 2009, 291.
18. Doll and Hill 1950.
19. Ibid., 746.
20. Cornfield 1951.
21. Sir Richard Peto had a copy of the questionnaire sent to me in an email dated April 16, 2009.
22. However, those who chose to answer were *not* representative of the total. They were in better health. But this effect of selection wore off after some years. Once the

less healthy doctors not participating in the study died, the participants became representative of all the doctors still alive. See Doll and Hill 1954.

23. To measure the risk of dying from lung cancer, a simple way would be to divide the number of cases by the number of doctors in each smoking category. The ten-year risk for never smokers would be 3/5,439, or 0.0055 per thousand. The problem is that not all doctors were followed for ten years. Some died from causes other than lung cancer, and it is not possible to know whether they would have developed lung cancer had they not died from another cause. For this reason, Doll and Hill calculated the number of *person-years* of exposure between 1951 and 1961; that is, they took the average of the numbers of survivors at the beginning and at the end of each year and summed them for the ten years of the study. For example, the number of male doctors ages forty-five to fifty-four was 7,117 on November 1, 1951, and 7,257 on November 1, 1952; thus, on average there were 7,187 ([7,117 + 7,257]/2) male doctors alive in that age group throughout that year. Similarly, there were, on average, 7,319 male doctors alive in the same age group throughout the second year, 7,366 throughout the third year, and 7,283 throughout the fourth year. The total number of years lived by male doctors in that age group was therefore calculated to be 29,155 years (7,187 + 7,319 + 7,366 + 7,283). Thus, the principle of person–time calculation is that subjects are replaced by the number of units of time they have been followed up while still at risk of developing the outcome of interest. A doctor for whom all vital information was available for the full ten years and who was still healthy in November 1961 would count for ten person-years, whereas another doctor who had been followed for two years but then died of any cause would count for two person-years. The total number of person-years is indicated in figure 7.3. The average duration of follow-up was 7.9 years (42,860/5,439) for the never smokers and 8.3 years (149,000/18,060) for ever smokers. Thus, smokers were followed up for a little bit longer than the nonsmokers.

24. 0.00007 × 45 = 0.00315, or 0.3 percent. There are more exact ways of computing long-term risks, but they can't be done offhand.

25. Doll et al. 2004.

26. Fisher 1959; Stolley 1991.

27. Fisher 1959, 46.

28. Schwartz et al. 1961.

29. There remained a problem in the French study, however: in the small subgroups of heavy smokers of thirty or more cigarettes per day, the lung cancer cases inhaled less than the noncancer controls. Did controls smoke just as many cigarettes as the lung cancer cases but leave longer butts? Did controls inhale so deeply that the potentially dangerous particles of tobacco smoke were deposited in the alveoli rather than in the bronchi? Such were the speculations by Doll and Hill, who modestly acknowledged in 1964 that "there are, of course, many facets to smoking of which we are ignorant" (Doll and Hill 1964, 1461).

30. Surgeon General's Advisory Committee 1964.
31. Kluger 1997, 242–244.
32. Surgeon General's Advisory Committee 1964, 31.
33. Brandt 2007, 296.
34. See Kluger 1997; Brandt 2007; Proctor 2012.
35. Rabin 2011.
36. Giovino et al. 2012.
37. See Morabia 2004a. According to the website studentscholarships.org, there are now about five thousand people employed as epidemiologists in the United States, and "over the next 10 years epidemiolog[y] will be one of the fastest growing occupations. They should experience a 13.6% rate of growth during this time period." There are about fifty schools of public health in the United States alone.

## 8. DAILY LIFE MYSTERIES AND EPIDEMIOLOGY

1. This story is recounted in Bastian 2004.
2. Moser 1956.
3. Moser 1959.
4. Moser 1969.
5. Feinstein 1967, 39.
6. Cochrane 1972, 70.
7. Cochrane 1979, quoted on the Cochrane Collaboration website, http://www.cochrane.org/about-us/history/archie-cochrane#REF2.
8. Cochrane 1989.
9. To find a Cochrane review, you need to use the link provided on the website http://www2.cochrane.org/reviews/. You can also go through the Cochrane Library website at http://www.thecochranelibrary.com/view/0/index.html. Abstracts are free, but the full reviews are sometimes at a cost. A fraction of the material exists in several languages.
10. Cochrane Collaboration, "About Us," http://www.cochrane.org/about-us, accessed September 9, 2013.
11. Pauker 1976; Sisson, Schoomaker, and Ross 1976; Weinstein 1980.
12. In the mid-1970s, clinical decision analysis was practiced only by a small group of clinical researchers. Their work gained respectability when it appeared in leading US medical journals such as the *Annals of Internal Medicine*, the *New England Journal of Medicine*, and the *Journal of the American Medical Association* as well as in textbooks.
13. Oxman, Sackett, and Guyatt 1993.
14. Sackett et al. 1996.
15. Petitti 2005.

16. Wegwarth et al. 2012; Morabia 2013c.
17. Screening tests are different from diagnostic tests. A good screening test, when it is negative, is interpreted as ruling out the disease, but most screening tests are not necessarily indicative of the presence of the disease when they are positive. Thus, a screenee is reassured and nothing more when the test is negative, but, if the test is positive, he or she has to undergo additional investigations that are more invasive and expensive than the screening test itself. For example, a positive mammogram is usually followed by a collection of mammary tissue using needle aspiration or biopsy. The majority of the aspirations and biopsies come back negative and rule out cancer in some patients. The minority of positive aspirations and biopsies are treated as real cancers.

## 9. IS THIS TREATMENT DANGEROUS FOR HEALTH?

1. "British Thalidomide Charity" 2012.
2. This story is related in the terrifying book *Dark Remedy: The Impact of Thalidomide and Its Revival as a Vital Medicine* (Stephens and Brynner 2001).
3. Ibid., 24.
4. McBride 1961.
5. Lee et al. 1983.
6. Vandenbroucke 2004.

## 10. DOES THE TREATMENT WORK?

1. Hrobjartsson, Gøtzsche, and Gluud 1998.
2. Therapeutic Trial Committee of the Medical Research Council 1934.
3. For a historical discussion of the discovery of the complementary roles of randomization and concealment of the randomization sequence, see Chalmers 2010.
4. In an analysis of the evolution of mortality in Geneva during the twentieth century, the mortality rate from tuberculosis in 1900 was 3 per 1,000 (Morabia 1996a). In 1900, 194 of every 100,000 US residents died from tuberculosis ("Achievements in Public Health" 1999).
5. Medical Research Council 1948.
6. Cochrane 1972, 11.
7. Quoted in Bastian 2004.
8. Kaptchuk 1998.
9. There exists a vast scientific literature on placebos, but I took these examples from a popular science article (Brown 1998).
10. Dimond, Kittle, and Crockett 1960.
11. Hrobjartsson and Gøtzsche 2001, 2010.

12. Kirsch et al. 2002.

13. Concorde Coordinating Committee 1994.

## 11. WHAT IS THE OPTIMAL MEDICAL DECISION?

1. Morabia et al. 1994.

2. Karim et al. 2010.

3. Centers for Disease Control and Prevention 2010c.

4. Exactly 28.6 women, which, rounded, is 29.

5. A handy way to compute the NNT is to take the inverse of the rate difference: NNT = 1/RD = 100 women/3.5 years = 28.6, which, rounded, is 29 women per year.

## 12. HEALTH RISK OR HEALTH BENEFIT?

1. Galea et al. 2011.

2. To understand the connection between the 1.8 and the 80 percent, consider two numbers, 1.8 and 1; if we subtract, 1.8 − 1.0 = 0.8, the 0.8 is 80 percent more than the 1, or 80 percent in excess. The same logic can be applied to the mortality rates and the excess mortality in our example.

3. A × B × C = 20% × 34.5% × 1.8 million = 124,200 deaths.

4. Multiple Risk Factor Intervention Trial Research Group 1982.

5. Rosborough et al. 1990.

6. ATBC: Alpha-Tocopherol 1994. See also Hennekens et al. 1996 and Omenn et al. 1996.

7. Daily doses were 120 milligrams of ascorbic acid (vitamin C), 30 milligrams of vitamin E, 6 milligrams of beta-carotene, 100 micrograms of selenium, and 20 milligrams of zinc (Hercberg et al. 2004).

8. To avoid unwarranted generalization, let me note that vitamin D, deficits of which are common and which is not an antioxidant, has multiple health benefits and a low toxicity among people in good health.

9. Willett et al. 1993.

10. Mozaffarian et al. 2006.

11. Angell et al. 2012.

12. Centers for Disease Control and Prevention 2012.

## 13. IS THIS SCREENING USEFUL?

1. Shapiro et al. 1988.

2. To randomize, the 62,000 women were listed by age, parity (number of fetal births), and occupation. Mammographic screening or usual care was then allocated

alternatively to each woman following the order of the list. In general, this systematic (alternating) allocation scheme does not create groups as comparable as a truly random allocation procedure would.

3. The mortality rate of 1.2 percent per year corresponds to a life expectancy of 100 years/1.2 = 83 years. The mortality rate of 1.3 percent per year corresponds to a life expectancy of 100 years/1.3 = 77 years. The number of years of life gained attributable to the screening is six years: 83 − 77 = 6.

4. In favor of mammographic screening, see Nelson et al. 2009; against, see Gøtzsche and Nielsen 2009.

5. In the European study, after nine years of follow-up, prostate cancer was diagnosed in 8.2 percent of the 72,890 men who were systematically screened for PSA and in 4.8 percent of the 89,353 men in the comparison group. There were 0.35 deaths from prostate cancer for 1,000 participants in the screened group versus 0.41 per 1,000 in the comparison group. To prevent one death from prostate cancer in the screened group, one would have to measure PSA and eventually perform complementary diagnostic tests in 1,410 men and treat 48 cancers. See Schroeder et al. 2009.

6. The PSA test is an inexpensive and noninvasive prostate cancer screening test, but, as the text indicates, it is difficult to interpret. The uncertainty associated with the test has been quantified. If the limit between normal and pathologic PSA is set to 4 nanograms per milliliters, there will be 50–80 percent false negatives and 7–10 percent false positives. This means that of 100 men who really have prostate cancer, 50 to 80 will be unwarrantedly told that they have no prostate cancer, and, of 100 men who really don't have prostate cancer, 7 to 10 will have to uselessly undergo invasive diagnostic tests such as a needle aspiration or a biopsy (Thompson et al. 2005). For cancer prostate screening to become effective, we need a better test than PSA, with less false negatives and more true positives, as well as an effective treatment.

7. Some urologists and oncologists believe that PSA screening has contributed to rarefying the proportion of advanced, incurable prostate cancers.

8. The results of the RCT comparing CT scan with chest X-ray in screening for lung cancer in heavy smokers were published in August 2011 (Aberle et al. 2011).

## 14. GROUP COMPARISONS ALSO FAIL

1. Jueni et al. 2004. It is, however, worse when dangerous drugs are commercialized without having been rigorously tested. See Moore 1995 about Tambocor, a drug that was prescribed for cardiac arrhythmias but that caused sudden deaths, an adverse effect finally demonstrated in an RCT.

2. Hymes et al. 1981.

3. Marmor et al. 1982; see also Morabia 1995.

4. Barré-Sinoussi et al. 1983.

5. Jaffe et al. 1983, 148.

6. Moore 1995.
7. Morabia 1992.
8. Michael Marmor and Neil Dubin (1990) reported that alternative analyses of their data yielded higher relative risks for sexual partners than for nitrite use. See also Vandenbroucke and Pardoel 1989.
9. Wilson 1966, cover blurb.
10. Ibid., 182–183.
11. Rossouw et al. 2002.
12. Progestin was conceivably responsible for the increased occurrence of coronary heart disease because a similar increase was not observed in the women who received estrogen only, not described here.
13. NNT = 10,000 women/7 per year = 1,429 women treated with replacement therapy per year to provoke one heart attack.
14. Morabia and Costanza 2006. For France, see Ringa et al. 2010.
15. Hernan et al. 2008.
16. Stampfer 2008.
17. Hoover 2008; Vandenbroucke 2009.


## 15. EPIDEMIOLOGIC LITERACY AND "EARTHLY SELF-REALIZATION"

1. The US Institute of Medicine has called for a greater epidemiologic literacy in the society at large (Committee on Educating Public Health Professionals for the 21st Century and Institute of Medicine of the National Academies 2003). Also see Riegelman 2008.
2. Fine, Goldacre, and Haines 2013, 1251.
3. Cole 2012.
4. The Swiss nongovernmental organization Health on the Net (HON, www.hon.ch) has the mission to promote the quality of health information available online. Medical and health websites abiding by the HON Code of Conduct can be identified by the HON logo.
5. Christen et al. 2011.
6. Fragment of a text published in *Die Umschau* in September 1946, then in *Erasme* in 1946, and quoted in *Le Monde*, April 16, 2000, my translation.
7. Fraser 1987, 309.
8. Kaelin et al. 2007.
9. Comparable issues exist for teaching mathematical skills. Linking math concepts to real-life applications has been proposed as a way of improving American students' performance on international math tests: "How often do most adults encounter a situation in which they need to solve a quadratic equation? Do they need to know what constitutes a 'group of transformations' or a 'complex number'? Of course

professional mathematicians, physicists and engineers need to know all this, but most citizens would be better served by studying how mortgages are priced, how computers are programmed and how the statistical results of a medical trial are to be understood" (Garfunkel and Mumford 2011).

10. Fogel 2004, 70.

11. Marks 1995, cited in Fogel 2004, 72.

12. This goal was for the thirty mostly Western countries grouped into the Organization for Economic Cooperation and Development, including the United States, the United Kingdom, Canada, and Australia, to name some English-speaking countries.

13. Fogel 2004, 79. Indeed, an increasing proportion of "older and wiser students" are attending universities. According to the National Center for Education Statistics, the number of graduate students older than fifty grew by 38 percent between 2001 and 2005, from about 125,000 to 173,000, more than twice the rate of growth for graduate students overall; at Johns Hopkins University, Dartmouth College, and the University of Oklahoma, at least 10 percent of the liberal arts graduate students are older than fifty-five or retired; at Harvard University Extension School, about 16 percent of 484 candidates for the master of liberal arts degree are older than fifty (Larson 2008). In the long run, the growing proportion of adults engaging in lifelong education will challenge the way education is provided because adults bring not only their curiosity and desire to understand themselves and their environment better, but also their life experience and experiential knowledge.

## 16. BEYOND EPIDEMIOLOGY

1. For example, Susser and Stein 2009 and Krieger 2011 describe the evolution of theories in which epidemiologists have embedded the design of group comparisons.

2. Elveback, Guillier, and Keating 1970.

3. This can also be an ambiguous definition of normality. The cholesterol data come from the follow-up of 320,000 middle-aged men examined as part of the MRFIT in the United States. It is legitimate to ponder whether the relation of their blood cholesterol levels to heart disease risk apply to the English male population and so on.

4. Kolata 2008.

5. This is the function of the national surveys of health, nutrition, and behavioral risk factor that exist in many countries.

6. Ledermann 1956.

7. Rose 1993.

8. Rose used the results from Intersalt, an international study conducted in fifty-two recruitment centers in thirty-two countries and involving 10,079 men and women ages twenty to fifty-nine. Besides the Yanomamo Indians of Brazil, there are thirty-two centers in Europe, including the United Kingdom and the countries of the former Soviet Union; seven in the Americas; eleven in Asia; and two in

Africa (Rose and Day 1990). Intersalt performed a detailed assessment of alcohol consumption over the previous week and over the previous twenty-four hours based on questionnaires followed by in-person interviews. The ethanol content of local beverages was determined in a laboratory. Three to four glasses of wine contain 34 grams of ethanol—that is, of pure alcohol (Marmot et al. 1994).

9. LaVallee, Williams, and Yi 2009.

10. Recent studies of the dynamic of behavior changes in populations tend to corroborate Ledermann and Rose's observations. Nicholas Christakis and James Fowler (2007) have tracked the evolution of behaviors within populations for which they had mapped the familial and amicable interpersonal connections beforehand: every person had identified relatives and friends. Christakis and Fowler then followed how weight evolved across several years. Apparently, overweight individuals popped up preferentially within subgroups of people personally connected. The main determinant of one's weight was not the behavior of a geographically close person—the neighbor, for example—but of someone who was within the individual's social network—the best friend, the brother, the sister, or the spouse. Weight gain seemed to be preceded by a change in social norm. The idea is that people are at greater risk of becoming overweight or obese when they belong to a social network that tolerates these conditions. Christakis and Fowler are proposing an attractive theory based on a creative mode of data analysis. A discussion of their work can be found in Johns 2010 and Gelman 2011.

11. Does it help you to know that a statistical test indicated that—assuming that the treatment was ineffective and that the same trial was done again in a new population—the probability of finding a difference as extreme or more extreme was 4 percent ($p = 0.04$)? A widely accepted convention is that an observed difference is considered not due to chance if $p$ is lower than 5 percent. I did not cover statistical tests in this book because they seem to me less important for the lay public than the validity of the comparisons and the magnitude of the observed differences. But Professor Goodman gives the $p$-value to his students.

12. Harris et al. 1999.

13. Letters to the editor and the study authors' responses were published in *Archives of Internal Medicine* 160 (2000): 1870–1878.

14. For example, Aviles et al. 2001.

## EPILOGUE: THE END OF EPIDEMIOLOGY?

1. Pinel 1807.

2. In practice, the methods and mathematics of the advocates of quantitative medicine were very basic. There were exceptions, such as the textbook of medical statistics by Jules Gavarret (Huth 2006), but in general nineteenth-century doctors used only means and proportions.

3. D'Amador 1837, 25.
4. See Morabia 2006.
5. Bernard [1865] 1957, 286, my translation.
6. Ibid., 282.
7. Ibid., 286.
8. Ibid., 134.
9. Ibid., 194, emphasis added.
10. Ibid., emphasis added.
11. Ibid.
12. Ibid.
13. Ibid., 214.
14. Ibid., 194.

## APPENDIX 3: WHY COHORT AND CASE–CONTROL STUDIES CONCUR

1. Another way to put it is: $1/1 \div \frac{1}{4} = 4$.
2. In chapter 7, I rounded the percentages to one decimal. Thus, $99.7/0.3 \div 95.8/4.2 = 14.6$.
3. The historical publications establishing and popularizing why cohort and case-control studies concur are Miettinen 1976, Greenland and Thomas 1982, and Rothman 1986. I realize that, overall, this section is difficult to understand upon the first read through. I have tried to be precise and explanatory. The second time around, it should make much more sense.

# BIBLIOGRAPHY

Aberle DR, Adams AM, Berg CD, Black WC, Clapp JD, Fagerstrom RM, Gareen IF, Gatsonis C, Marcus PM, Sicks JD. 2011. Reduced lung-cancer mortality with low-dose computed tomographic screening. *New England Journal of Medicine* 365:395–409.

Achievements in public health, 1900–1999: Control of infectious diseases. 1999. *Morbidity and Mortality Weekly Report* 48:621–629.

Ackerknecht EH. 1967. *Medicine at the Paris Hospital, 1794–1848.* Baltimore: John Hopkins University Press.

Ackerknecht EH. 1986. *La Médecine hospitalière à Paris (1794–1848).* Paris: Payot.

Alzheimer's gene "linked to vitamin D." 2011. *Telegraph,* May 30.

Angell SY, Cobb LK, Curtis CJ, Konty KJ, Silver LD. 2012. Change in trans fatty acid content of fast-food purchases associated with New York City's restaurant regulation: A pre–post study. *Annals of Internal Medicine* 157:81–86.

Anda RF, Williamson DF, Escobedo LG, Remington PL, Mast EE, Madans JH. 1992. Self-perceived stress and the risk of peptic ulcer disease: A longitudinal study of US adults. *Archives of Internal Medicine* 152:829–833.

Appleby A. 1980. The disappearance of plague: A continuing puzzle. *Economic History Review* 33:161–173.

ATBC: Alpha-Tocopherol B-CCPSG. 1994. The effect of vitamin E and beta-carotene on the incidence of lung cancer and other cancers in male smokers. *New England Journal of Medicine* 330:1029–1035.

Aviles JM, Whelan SE, Hernke DA, Williams BA, Kenny KE, O'Fallon WM, Kopecky SL. 2001. Intercessory prayer and cardiovascular disease progression in a coronary care unit population: a randomized controlled trial. *Mayo Clinic Proceedings* 76:1192–1198.

Bailey, RC. 1991. *The Behavioral Ecology of Efe Pygmy Men in the Ituri Forest, Zaire.* Anthropological Papers no. 86. Ann Harbor: Museum of Anthropology, University of Michigan.

Barré-Sinoussi F, Chermann JC, Rey F, Nugeyre MT, Chamaret S, Gruest J, Dauguet C, Axler-Blin C, Vezinet-Brun F, Rouzioux C, Rozenbaum W, Montagnier L. 1983. Isolation of a T-lymphotropic retrovirus from a patient at risk for acquired immune deficiency syndrome (AIDS). *Science* 220:868–871.

Barry JM. 2005. *The Great Influenza: The Epic Story of the Deadliest Plague in History*. New York: Penguin.

Bartley H. 1832. *Illustrations of Cholera Asphyxia in Its Different Stages Selected from Cases Treated at the Cholera Hospital, Rivington Street*. New York: Jackson.

Bastian H. 2004. *Down and Almost Out in Scotland: George Orwell, Tuberculosis, and Getting Streptomycin in 1948*. James Lind Library. http://www.jameslindlibrary.org/illustrating/articles/down-and-almost-out-in-scotland-george-orwell-tuberculosis-and. Accessed September 19, 2013.

Benedictow O. 2006. *The Black Death 1346–1353: The Complete History*. Cambridge: Brewer.

Bernard C. [1865] 1957. *An Introduction to the Study of Experimental Medicine*. New York: Dover.

Biraben J. 1975. *Les hommes et la peste en France et dans les pays européens et méditerranéens (Civilisations et sociétés)*. Paris: Mouton.

Black W. 1789. *Arithmetickal and Medical Analysis of the Diseases and Mortality of the Human Species*. London: Dilly.

Bollet AJ. 1992. Politics and pellagra: The epidemic of pellagra in the U.S. in the early twentieth century. *Yale Journal of Biological Medicine* 65:211–221.

Boston Collaborative Drug Surveillance Group. 1974. Regular aspirin intake and acute myocardial infarction. *British Medical Journal* 1:440–443.

Bown SR. 2003. *Scurvy: How a Surgeon, a Mariner, and a Gentleman Solved the Greatest Medical Mystery of the Age of Sail*. New York: Dunne.

Boylston A. 2012. *Defying Providence: Smallpox and the Forgotten 18th Century Medical Revolution*. North Charleston, SC: CreateSpace Independent Publishing Platform.

Brandt A. 2007. *The Cigarette Century: The Rise, Fall, and Deadly Persistence of the Product That Defined America*. New York: Perseus.

British thalidomide charity rebuffs Gruenenthal Group's apology. 2012. *Huffington Post*, August 31. http://www.huffingtonpost.co.uk/2012/08/31/british-thalidomide-charity-drug-company-_n_1847670.html.

Brody, Jane E. 1996. In smoking, study sees risk of cancer of the breast. *New York Times*, May 6.

Brown WA. 1998. The placebo effect. *Scientific American* 278:90–95.

Buchholz U, Bernard H, Werber D, Bohmer MM, Remschmidt C, Wilking H, Deleré Y, an der Heiden M, Adlhoch C, Dreesman J, Ehlers J, Ethelberg S, Faber M, Frank C, Fricke G, Greiner M, Hohle M, Ivarsson S, Jark U, Kirchner M, Koch J, Krause G, Luber P, Rosner B, Stark K, Kuhne M. 2011. German outbreak of *Escherichia coli* O104:H4 associated with sprouts. *New England Journal of Medicine* 365:1763–1770.

Bulstrode HT. 1902. Report upon alleged oyster-borne enteric fever and other illness following the mayoral banquets at Winchester and Southampton, and upon enteric fever occurring simultaneously elsewhere, and also ascribed to oysters. Medical Officer's Annual Report to Local Government Board. *British Parliamentary Papers* 26:129–179.

Cancer of the lung. 1942. *British Medical Journal* 1:672–673.

Cancer of the lung. 1952. *Lancet* 2:667.

Carpenter KJ. 1986. *The History of Scurvy and Vitamin C.* Cambridge: Cambridge University Press.

Carpenter, KJ. 2004. The Nobel Prize and the discovery of vitamins. http://nobelprize. org/nobel_prizes/medicine/articles/carpenter/index.html.

Carter KC. 1983. *Ignaz Semmelweis: The Etiology, Concept, and Prophylaxis of Childbed Fever.* Madison: University of Wisconsin Press.

Carter K, Carter B. 2005. *Childbed Fever. A Scientific Biography of Ignaz Semmelweis.* New Brunswick, NJ: Transaction.

Centers for Disease Control and Prevention. 2010a. 2009 H1N1: Overview of a pandemic. Updated December 9. http://www.cdc.gov/h1n1flu/yearinreview/yir5.htm.

Centers for Disease Control and Prevention. 2010b. The 2009 H1N1 pandemic: Summary highlights, April 2009–April 2010. Updated June 16. http://www.cdc.gov/ h1n1flu/cdcresponse.htm.

Centers for Disease Control and Prevention. 2010c. CDC statement on CAPRISA microbicide study results. July 19. http://www.cdc.gov/nchhstp/newsroom/CAPRI-SAMediaStatement.html.

Centers for Disease Control and Prevention. 2011. Final estimates for 2009–10 seasonal influenza and influenza A (H1N1) 2009 monovalent vaccination coverage—United States, August 2009 through May 2010. Updated May 13. http://www.cdc.gov/flu/ professionals/vaccination/coverage_0910estimates.htm.

Centers for Disease Control and Prevention. 2012. Trans Fat: The Facts. Updated April 12. http://www.cdc.gov/nutrition/everyone/basics/fat/transfat.html.

Chalmers I. 2010. Why the 1948 MRC trial of streptomycin used treatment allocation based on random numbers. JLL Bulletin: Commentaries on the history of treatment evaluation. James Lind Library.http://www.jameslindlibrary.org/illustrating/ articles/why-the-1948-mrc-trial-of-streptomycin-used-treatment-allocation, accessed September 19, 2013.

Christakis NA, Fowler JH. 2007. The spread of obesity in a large social network over 32 years. *New England Journal of Medicine* 357:370–378.

Christen WG, Schaumberg DA, Glynn RJ, Buring JE. 2011. Dietary ω-3 fatty acid and fish intake and incident age-related macular degeneration in women. *Archives of Ophthalmology* 129:921–929.

Cochrane AL. 1972. *Effectiveness and Efficiency: Random Reflections on Health Services.* London: Nuffield Provincial Hospitals Trust.

Cochrane AL. 1979. 1931–1971: A critical review, with particular reference to the medical profession. In G Feeling-Smith and N Wells, eds., *Medicines for the Year 2000*, 1–11. London: Office of Health Economics.

Cochrane, AL. 1989. Foreword in I Chalmers, M Enkin, MJNC Keirse, eds., *Effective Care in Pregnancy and Childbirth.* Oxford: Oxford University Press. http:// www.jameslindlibrary.org/illustrating/records/effective-care-in-pregnancy-and-childbirth/key_passages.

Cohen M, Armalagos G. 1984. *Paleopathology at the Origin of Agriculture*. New York: Academic Press.

Cole A. 2012. Disease sleuths surf for outbreaks online. NPR, February 24. http://www.npr.org/blogs/health/2012/02/07/146519243/disease-sleuths-surf-for-outbreaks-online.

Committee on Educating Public Health Professionals for the 21st Century and Institute of Medicine of the National Academies. 2003. *Who Will Keep the Public Healthy? Educating Public Health Professionals for the 21st Century*. Washington, DC: National Academies Press.

Concorde Coordinating Committee. 1994. MRC/ANRS randomised double-blind controlled trial of immediate and deferred Zidovudine in symptom-free HIV infection. *Lancet* 343:871–881.

Continuing fight. 1949. *Time*, March 7. http://content.time.com/time/magazine/article/0,9171,853667,00.html.

Cornfield J. 1951. A method of estimating comparative rates from clinical data: Applications to cancer of the lung, breast, and cervix. *Journal of the National Cancer Institute* 11:1269–1275.

Council of Europe Parliamentary Assembly. 2010. *The Handling of the H1N1 Pandemic: More Transparency Needed*. 2010. N.p.: Council of Europe Parliamentary Assembly.

Crow JF. 1999. Hardy, Weinberg, and language impediments. *Genetics* 152:821–825.

De Montellano BR. 1990. *Aztec Medicine, Health, and Nutrition*. New Brunswick, NJ: Rutgers University Press.

Descartes R. 1953. *Oeuvres et lettres*. Ed. André Bridoux. Paris: Gallimard.

Diamond J. 1999. *Guns, Germs, and Steel: The Fates of Human Societies*. New York: Norton.

Diesel engine exhaust causes lung cancer, WHO agency says. 2012. *Bloomberg*, June 12. http://www.bloomberg.com/news/2012-06-12/diesel-engine-exhaust-causes-lung-cancer-who-agency-says.html.

Diet: Eating fish found to ward off eye disease. 2011. *New York Times*, March 22.

Dimond EG, Kittle CF, Crockett JE. 1960. Comparison of internal mammary artery ligation and sham operation for angina pectoris. *American Journal of Cardiology* 5:483–486.

Doll R, Hill AB. 1950. Smoking and carcinoma of the lung: Preliminary report. *British Medical Journal* 2:739–748.

Doll R, Hill AB. 1954. The mortality of doctors in relation to their smoking habits; a preliminary report. *British Medical Journal* 2:1451–1455.

Doll R, Hill AB. 1964. Mortality in relation to smoking: Ten years' observations of British doctors. *British Medical Journal* 1:1399–1410, 1460–1467.

Doll R, Peto R, Boreham J, Sutherland I. 2004. Mortality in relation to smoking: 50 years' observations on male British doctors. *British Medical Journal* 328:1519–1528.

Donaldson IML. 2013. A mid-seventeeth-century defence of Galenism. *Journal of the Royal College of Physicians of Edinburgh* 43:88–90.

Donoghue HD, Marcsik A, Matheson C, Vernon K, Nuorala E, Molto JE, Greenblatt CL, Spigelman M. 2005. Co-infection of *Mycobacterium tuberculosis* and *Mycobacterium leprae* in human archaeological samples: A possible explanation for the historical decline of leprosy. *Proceedings of the Royal Society B: Biological Sciences* 272:389–394.

Durand JD. 1960. The population statistics of China, A.D. 2–1953. *Population Studies* 13:209–256.

Elveback LR, Guillier CL, Keating FR, Jr. 1970. Health, normality, and the ghost of Gauss. *Journal of the American Medical Association* 211:69–75.

English J, Willius F, Berkson J. 1940. Tobacco and coronary disease. *Journal of the American Medical Association* 115:1327–1328.

The etiology of pellagra. 1914. *Journal of the American Medical Association* 13:1114–1115.

Evans R. 2005. *Death in Hamburg: Society and Politics in the Cholera Years.* London: Penguin.

Fairchild AL, Oppenheimer GM. 1998. Public health nihilism vs pragmatism: History, politics, and the control of tuberculosis. *American Journal of Public Health* 88:1105–1117.

Feinstein AR. 1967. *Clinical Judgment.* Baltimore: Williams and Wilkins.

Fenner F. 1970. The effect of changing social organization on the infectious diseases of man. In SV Boyden, ed., *The Impact of Civilization on the Biology of Man,* 48–68. Toronto: University of Toronto Press.

Fine P, Goldacre B, Haines A. 2013. Epidemiology—a science for the people. *Lancet* 381:1249–1252.

Fisher R. 1959. *Smoking: The Cancer Controversy. Some Attempts to Assess the Evidence.* Edinburgh: Oliver and Boyd.

Fogel RW. 2004. *The Escape from Hunger and Premature Death, 1700–2100.* Cambridge: Cambridge University Press.

Frank J. 1788. *System einer vollstaendigen medicinischen Polizey.* Mannheim, Germany: Schwan & Gotz.

Frank J. 1790. De populorum miseria, morborum genetrice. *Delectus Opusculorum Medicorum* ix:305–324.

Fraser DW. 1987. Epidemiology as a liberal art. *New England Journal of Medicine* 316:309–314.

Galea S, Tracy M, Hoggatt KJ, Dimaggio C, Karpati A. 2011. Estimated deaths attributable to social factors in the United States. *American Journal of Public Health* 101:1456–1465.

Garfunkel S, Mumford D. 2011. How to fix our math education. *New York Times,* August 24.

Gelman A. 2011. Controversy over the Christakis–Fowler findings on the contagion of obesity. *The Monkey Cage,* June 10. http://themonkeycage.org/2011/06/10/1-lyonss-statistical-critiques-seem-reasonable-to-me-there-could-well-be-something-important-that-im-missing-but-until-i-hear-otherwise-for-example-in-a-convincing-reply-by-christakis-and-f/.

Giovino GA, Mirza SA, Samet JM, Gupta PC, Jarvis MJ, Bhala N, Peto R, Zatonski W, Hsia J, Morton J, Palipudi KM, Asma S. 2012. Tobacco use in 3 billion individuals from 16 countries: An analysis of nationally representative cross-sectional household surveys. *Lancet* 380:668–679.

Goldberger J, Waring C, Tanner W. 1923. Pellagra prevention by diet among institutional inmates. *Public Health Reports* 38:2361–2368.

Goldberger J, Waring C, Willets D. 1915. A test of diet in the prevention of pellagra. *Public Health Reports* 30:3117–3131.

Goldberger J, Wheeler GA, Sydenstricker E. 1920. A study of the relation of family income and other economic factors to pellagra incidence in seven cotton-mill villages of South Carolina in 1916. *Public Health Reports* 35:2673–2714.

Good week for people who make their grievances heard at work. 2011. *The Australian*, May 28.

Gottfried R. 1983. *The Black Death: Natural and Human Disaster in Medieval Europe.* New York: Free Press.

Gøtzsche PC, Nielsen M. 2009. Screening for breast cancer with mammography. *Cochrane Database Systematic Reviews* 4:CD001877.

Graunt, J. [1662] 2004. *Natural and Political Observations Made Upon the Bills of Mortality.* Baltimore: Johns Hopkins University Press. http://www.ac.wwu.edu/~stephan/Graunt/.

Greenland S, Thomas DC. 1982. On the need for the rare disease assumption in case-control studies. *American Journal of Epidemiology* 116:547–553.

Hamlin C. 1985. Providence and putrefaction: Victorian sanitarians and the natural theology of health and disease. *Victorian Studies* 28:381–411.

Hardy A. 2003a. Commentary: Bread and alum, syphilis and sunlight. Rickets in the nineteenth century. *International Journal of Epidemiology* 32:337–340.

Hardy A. 2003b. Exorcizing Molly Malone: Typhoid and shellfish consumption in urban Britain 1860–1960. *History Workshop Journal* 55:73–90.

Harper KN, Ocampo PS, Steiner BM, George RW, Silverman MS, Bolotin S, Pillay A, Saunders NJ, Armelagos GJ. 2008. On the origin of the treponematoses: A phylogenetic approach. *PLIS Neglected Tropical Diseases* 2:e148.

Harris WS, Gowda M, Kolb JW, Strychacz CP, Vacek JL, Jones PG, Forker A, O'Keefe JH, McCallister BD. 1999. A randomized, controlled trial of the effects of remote, intercessory prayer on outcomes in patients admitted to the coronary care unit. *Archives of Internal Medicine* 159:2273–2278.

Hennekens CH, Buring JE, Manson JE, Stampfer M, Rosner B, Cook NR, Belanger C, LaMotte F, Gaziano JM, Ridker PM, Willett W, Peto R. 1996. Lack of effect of long-term supplementation with beta carotene on the incidence of malignant neoplasms and cardiovascular disease. *New England Journal of Medicine* 334:1145–1149.

Hercberg S, Galan P, Preziosi P, Bertrais S, Mennen L, Malvy D, Roussel AM, Favier A, Briancon S. 2004. The SU.VI.MAX study: A randomized, placebo-controlled trial of the health effects of antioxidant vitamins and minerals. *Archives of Internal Medicine* 164:2335–2342.

Hernan MA, Alonso A, Logan R, Grodstein F, Michels KB, Willett WC, Manson JE, Robins JM. 2008. Observational studies analyzed like randomized experiments: An application to postmenopausal hormone therapy and coronary heart disease. *Epidemiology* 19:766–779.

Hill K, Hurtado AM. 1996. *Ache Life History: The Ecology and Demography of a Foraging People.* New York: De Gruyter.

Hoffman FL. 1931. Cancer and smoking habits. *Annals of Surgery* 93:50–67.

Hope, J. 2010. Walking six miles each week could reduce chances of getting Alzheimer's. *Daily Mail*, November 29. http://www.dailymail.co.uk/health/article-1334006/Alzheimers-disease-Walking-6-miles-week-reduce-risk.html#ixzz1Nqjm3wX1.

Hopkins D. 2002. *The Greatest Killer: Smallpox in History.* Chicago: University of Chicago Press.

Hoover RN. 2008. The sound and the fury: Was it all worth it? *Epidemiology* 19:780–782.

Hrobjartsson A, Gøtzsche PC. 2001. Is the placebo powerless? An analysis of clinical trials comparing placebo with no treatment. *New England Journal of Medicine* 344:1594–1602.

Hrobjartsson A, Gøtzsche PC. 2010. Placebo interventions for all clinical conditions. *Cochrane Database System Reviews* 1:CD003974.

Hrobjartsson A, Gøtzsche PC, Gluud C. 1998. The controlled clinical trial turns 100 years: Fibiger's trial of serum treatment of diphtheria. *British Medical Journal* 317:1243–1245.

Huth EJ. 2006. Jules Gavarret's *Principes généraux de statistique médicale*: A pioneering text on the statistical analysis of the results of treatments. James Lind Library. http://www.jameslindlibrary.org/illustrating/articles/jules-gavarrets-principes-generaux-de-statistique-medicale-a-p. Accessed September 19, 2013.

Hymes KB, Cheung T, Greene JB, Prose NS, Marcus A, Ballard H, William DC, Laubenstein LJ. 1981. Kaposi's sarcoma in homosexual men: A report of eight cases. *Lancet* 2:598–600.

The increase in cancer of the lung. 1932. *Lancet* 219:1206–1207.

Ingalls A. 1936. If you smoke. *Scientific American* 154:310–313.

Jaffe HW, Choi K, Thomas PA, Haverkos HW, Auerbach DM, Guinan ME, Rogers MF, Spira TJ, Darrow WW, Kramer MA, Friedman SM, Monroe JM, Friedman-Kien AE, Laubenstein LJ, Marmor M, Safai B, Dritz SK, Crispi SJ, Fannin SL, Orkwis JP, Kelter A, Rushing WR, Thacker SB, Curran JW. 1983. National case-control study of Kaposi's sarcoma and *Pneumocystis carinii* pneumonia in homosexual men: Part 1. Epidemiologic results. *Annals of Internal Medicine* 99:145–151.

Jefferson, T. 2010. Influenzae statement. Cochrane Collaboration. http://assembly.coe.int/CommitteeDocs/2010/Jefferson_statement.pdf.

Jefferson T, Di PC, Al-Ansary LA, Ferroni E, Thorning S, Thomas RE. 2010. Vaccines for preventing influenza in the elderly. *Cochrane Database Systematic Reviews* 2:CD004876.

Jefferson T, Di PC, Rivetti A, Bawazeer GA, Al-Ansary LA, Ferroni E. 2010. Vaccines for preventing influenza in healthy adults. *Cochrane Database Systematic Reviews* 7:CD001269.

Johns D. 2010. Everything is contagious. *Slate,* April 7. http://www.slate.com/articles/health_and_science/science/features/2010/everything_is_contagious/has_a_plague_of_social_illness_struck_mankind.html.

Johnson WM. 1929. Tobacco smoking: A clinical study. *Jounal of the American Medical Association* 93:665–667.

Jouanna J. 2001. *Hippocrates (Medicine and Culture).* Baltimore: Johns Hopkins University Press.

Jueni P, Nartey L, Reichenbach S, Sterchi R, Dieppe PA, Egger M. 2004. Risk of cardiovascular events and rofecoxib: Cumulative meta-analysis. *Lancet* 364:2021–2029.

Kaelin MA, Huebner WW, Nicolich MJ, Kimbrough ML. 2007. Field test of an epidemiology curriculum for middle school students. *American Journal of Health Education* 38:16–31.

Kaptchuk TJ. 1998. Powerful placebo: The dark side of the randomised controlled trial. *Lancet* 351:1722–1725.

Karim QA, Karim SS, Frohlich JA, Grobler AC, Baxter C, Mansoor LE, Kharsany AB, Sibeko S, Mlisana KP, Omar Z, Gengiah TN, Maarschalk S, Arulappan N, Mlotshwa M, Morris L, Taylor D. 2010. Effectiveness and safety of tenofovir gel, an antiretroviral microbicide, for the prevention of HIV infection in women. *Science* 329:1168–1174.

Keating C. 2009. *Smoking Kills: The Revolutionary Life of Richard Doll.* Oxford: Signal Books.

Kelly RL. 1995. *The Foraging Spectrum.* Washington, DC: Smithsonian Institution Press.

Kirkey S. 2011. Study shows caffeine might prevent pregnancy. *Ottawa Citizen,* May 25. http://forum.psychlinks.ca/pregnancy-infertility-newborns-toddlers/26497-new-study-shows-how-caffeine-might-prevent-pregnancy.html.

Kirsch, I, Moore T, Scoboria A, Nicholls S. 2002. The emperor's new drugs: An analysis of antidepressant medication data submitted to the U.S. Food and Drug Administration. *Prevention & Treatment* 5:1–17.

Kluger R. 1997. *Ashes to Ashes: America's Hundred-Year Cigarette War, the Public Health, and the Unabashed Triumph of Philip Morris.* New York: Vintage.

Kolata G. 2008. A study revives a debate on arthritis knee surgery. *New York Times,* September 10.

Kraut A. 2003. *Goldberger's War: The Life and Work of a Public Health Crusader.* New York: Hill and Wang.

Krieger N. 2011. *Epidemiology and the People's Health: Theory and Context.* New York: Oxford University Press.

Lane-Claypon, J. 1926. *A Further Report on Cancer of the Breast: Reports on Public Health and Medical Subjects*. Ministry of Health. London: His Majesty's Stationary Office.

Larson C. 2008. Older, and wiser, students. *New York Times*, October 22.

LaVallee RA, Williams GD, and Yi H. 2009. *Surveillance Report #87: Apparent per Capita Alcohol Consumption: National, State, and Regional Trends, 1970–2007*. Bethesda, MD: National Institute on Alcohol Abuse and Alcoholism, Division of Epidemiology and Prevention Research. http://alcoholism.about.com/gi/o.htm?zi=1/XJ&zT i=1&sdn=alcoholism&cdn=health&tm=6&f=00&su=p284.9.336.ip_p1026.7.336. ip_&tt=2&bt=0&bts=0&zu=http%3A//www.niaaa.nih.gov/Resources/DatabaseResources/QuickFacts/AlcoholSales/consum03.htm.

Ledermann S. 1956. *Alcool, alcoolisme, alcoolisation*. Paris: INED.

Lee NC, Rubin GL, Ory HW, Burkman RT. 1983. Type of intrauterine device and the risk of pelvic inflammatory disease. *Obstetrics & Gynecology* 62:1–6.

Leonhardt, D. 2009. After the Great Recession: Interview of President Obama. *New York Times*, April 28. http://www.nytimes.com/2009/05/03/magazine/03Obama-t. html?pagewanted=1&_r=1.

Levin M, Goldstein H, Gerhardt P. 1950. Cancer and tobacco smoking: A preliminary report. *Journal of the American Medical Association* 143:336–338.

Lilienfeld A, Lilienfeld D. 1980. The French influence on the development of epidemiology. In A Lilienfeld, ed., *Times, Places, and Persons: Aspects of the History of Epidemiology*, 28–42. Baltimore: Johns Hopkins University Press.

Lind J. 1753. *A Treatise of Scurvy*. Edinburgh: Edinburgh University Press.

Louis PCA. 1825. *Recherches anatomico-pathologiques sur la phthisie par PCA Louis*. Paris: Gabon.

Louis PCA. 1828. Recherche sur les effets de la saignée dans plusieurs maladies inflammatoires. *Archives générales de médecine* 18:321–336.

Louis PCA. 1835. *Recherches sur les effets de la saignée dans quelques maladies inflammatoires, et sur l'action de l'émétique et des vésicatoires dans la pneumonie*. Paris: Baillière.

Louis PCA. 1836. *Researches on the Effects of Bloodletting in Some Inflammatory Diseases Together with Researches on Phthisis*. Boston: Hilliard, Gray.

Louis PCA. 1841. *Recherches anatomiques, pathologiques et thérapeutiques sur la maladie connue sous les noms de gastro-entérite, fièvre putride, adynamique, ataxique, typhoïde, etc., comparée avec les maladies aiguës les plus ordinaires*. Deuxième éditon considérablement augmentée. 2 vol. Paris: Baillière.

Mann C. 2006. *1492: New Revelations of the Americas Before Columbus*. New York: Vintage.

Manson JE. 2010. Great health news for every woman! Plus, advice from Harvard University's JoAnn E. Manson, M.D. *Glamour*, June.

Marks HM. 1995. Revisiting "the origins of compulsory drug prescriptions." *American Journal of Public Health* 85:109–115.

Marks HM. 2003. Epidemiologists explain pellagra: Gender, race, and political economy in the work of Edgar Sydenstricker. *Journal of the History of Medicine* 58:34–55.

Marmor M, Dubin N. 1990. Re: "An autopsy of epidemiologic methods: the case of 'poppers' in the early epidemic of the acquired immunodeficiency syndrome (AIDS)." *American Journal of Epidemiology* 131:195–196.

Marmor M, Friedman-Kien AE, Laubenstein L, Byrum RD, William DC, D'onofrio S, Dubin N. 1982. Risk factors for Kaposi's sarcoma in homosexual men. *Lancet* 1:1083–1087.

Marmot MG, Elliott P, Shipley MJ, Dyer AR, Ueshima H, Beevers DG, Stamler R, Kesteloot H, Rose G, Stamler J. 1994. Alcohol and blood pressure: The INTERSALT study. *British Medical Journal* 308:1263–1267.

Martin PM, Martin-Granel E. 2006. 2,500-year evolution of the term epidemic. *Emerging Infectious Diseases* 12:976–980.

McAlonan E. 2008. This week: Banish puffy eyes. *Mail Online: Beauty Confidential,* April 30.

McBride WG. 1961. Thalidomide and congenital abnormalities. *Lancet* 278:1358.

McNeill W. 1977. *Plagues and People.* New York: Anchor Books.

Medical Research Council. 1948. Streptomycin treatment of pulmonary tuberculosis. *British Medical Journal* 2:769–782.

Medicine and health: Epidemiology. n.d. WWW Virtual Library. http://www.epibiostat. ucsf.edu/epidem/epidem.html. Accessed September 20, 2013.

Miettinen O. 1976. Estimability and estimation in case-referent studies. *American Journal of Epidemiology* 103:226–235.

Mill JS. 1882. On the composition of causes. In *A System of Logic Ratiocinative and Inductive,* 457–466. New York: Harper.

Miura M, Daynard RA, Samet JM. 2006. The role of litigation in tobacco control. *Salud Pública de Mexico* 48, Supplement 1:S121–S136.

Moore TJ. 1995. *Deadly Medicine: Why Tens of Thousands of Heart Patients Died in America's Worst Drug Disaster.* New York: Simon & Schuster.

Morabia A. 1992. Confounding in epidemiological studies. *British Medical Journal* 305:1225–1226.

Morabia A. 1995. Poppers, Kaposi's sarcoma, and HIV infection: Empirical example of a strong confounding effect? *Preventive Medicine* 24:90–95.

Morabia A. 1996a. Major causes of deaths between 1901 and 1990 in Geneva, Switzerland. *Sozial und Praeventivmedizin* 41:315–321.

Morabia A. 1996b. P. C. A. Louis and the birth of clinical epidemiology. *Journal of Clinical Epidemiology* 49:1327–1333.

Morabia A. 2004a. *History of Epidemiological Methods and Concepts.* Basel: Birkhaeuser.

Morabia, A. 2004b. Pierre-Charles-Alexandre Louis and the evaluation of bloodletting. James Lind Library. http://www.jameslindlibrary.org/illustrating/articles/ pierre-charles-alexandre-louis-and-the-evaluation-of-bloodletting.

Morabia A. 2005. *Le Bus Santé: Une aventure genevoise.* Geneva: Éditions Médecine et Hygiène.

Morabia A. 2006. Claude Bernard was a 19th century proponent of medicine based on evidence. *Journal of Clinical Epidemiology* 59:1150–1154.

Morabia A. 2007. Epidemiologic interactions, complexity, and the lonesome death of Max von Pettenkofer. *American Journal of Epidemiology* 166:1233–1238.

Morabia A. 2008a. Joseph Goldberger's research on the prevention of pellagra. *Journal of the Royal Society of Medicine* 101:566–568.

Morabia A. 2008b. Morabia responds to Wildner and Hofman about "The Context and Challenge of von Pettenkofer's Contributions." *American Journal of Epidemiology* 168:119–121.

Morabia A. 2009a. Epidemic and population patterns in the Chinese Empire (243 B.C.E. to 1911 C.E.): Quantitative analysis of a unique but neglected epidemic catalogue. *Epidemiology and Infection* 137:1361–1368.

Morabia A. 2009b. In defense of Pierre Louis who pioneered the epidemiological approach to good medicine. *Journal of Clinical Epidemiology* 62:1–5.

Morabia A. 2010. Janet Lane-Claypon: Interphase epitome. *Epidemiology* 21:573–576.

Morabia A. 2012. Quality, originality, and significance of the 1939 "Tobacco consumption and lung carcinoma" article by Mueller, including translation of a section of the paper. *Preventive Medicine* 55:171–177.

Morabia A. 2013a. Epidemiology's 350th anniversary: 1662–2012. *Epidemiology* 24:179–183.

Morabia A. 2013b. "Lung cancer and tobacco consumption": Technical evaluation of the 1943 paper by Schairer and Schoeniger published in Nazi Germany. *Journal of Epidemiology and Community Health* 67:208–212.

Morabia A. 2013c. Primary care physicians surveyed in this study mistakenly interpreted improved survival and increased detection with screening as evidence that screening saves lives. *Evidence-Based Medicine* 18:e6.

Morabia A, Bernstein M, Heritier S, Khatchatrian N. 1996. Relation of breast cancer with passive and active exposure to tobacco smoke. *American Journal of Epidemiology* 143:918–928.

Morabia A, Costanza MC. 2006. Recent reversal of trends in hormone therapy use in a European population. *Menopause* 13:111–115.

Morabia A, Guthold R. 2007. Wilhelm Weinberg's 1913 large retrospective cohort study: A rediscovery. *American Journal of Epidemiology* 165:727–733.

Morabia A, Hardy A. 2005. Oysters and enteric fever aetiology in 1900 England. *Journal of Epidemiology and Community Health* 59:100.

Morabia A, Rochat T. 2001. Reproducibility of Louis' definition of pneumonia. *Lancet* 358:1188.

Morabia A, Rubenstein B, Victora CG. 2013. Epidemiology and public health in 1906 England: Arthur Newsholme's methodological innovation to study breastfeeding and fatal diarrhea. *American Journal of Public Health* 103:e17–e22.

Morabia A, Steinig-Stamm M, Unger PF, Slosman D, Schneider PA, Perrier A, Junod AF. 1994. Applicability of decision analysis to everyday clinical practice: A controlled feasibility trial. *Journal of General Internal Medicine* 9:496–502.

Moser RH. 1956. Diseases of medical progress. *New England Journal of Medicine* 255:606–614.

Moser RH. 1959. *Diseases of Medical Progress.* Springfield, IL: Thomas.

Moser RH. 1969. *Diseases of Medical Progress: A Study of Iatrogenic Diseases.* Springfield, IL: Thomas.

Mote FW. 1999. *Imperial China, 900–1800.* Cambridge, MA: Harvard University Press.

Mozaffarian D, Katan MB, Ascherio A, Stampfer MJ, Willett WC. 2006. Trans fatty acids and cardiovascular disease. *New England Journal of Medicine* 354:1601–1613.

Mueller F. 1939. Tabakmissbrauch und Lungencarcinom. *Zeitschrift fuer Krebsforschung* 49:57–85.

Multiple Risk Factor Intervention Trial Research Group. 1982. Multiple risk factor intervention trial: Risk factor changes and mortality results. *Journal of the American Medical Association* 248:1465–1477.

Needham J. 1981. *Science in Traditional China.* Cambridge, MA: Harvard University Press.

Nelson HD, Tyne K, Naik A, Bougatsos C, Chan BK, Humphrey L. 2009. Screening for breast cancer: An update for the U.S. Preventive Services Task Force. *Annals of Internal Medicine* 151:727–742.

Noakes TD, Borresen J, Hew-Butler T, Lambert MI, Jordaan E. 2008. Semmelweis and the aetiology of puerperal sepsis 160 years on: An historical review. *Epidemiology and Infection* 136:1–9.

Nutton V. 1983. The seeds of disease: An explanation of contagion and infection from the Greeks to the Renaissance. *Medical History* 27:1–34.

Ochsner A, DeBakey M. 1939. Primary pulmonary malignancy: Treatment by total pneumonectomy. *Surgery, Gynecology, and Obstetrics* 68:435–451.

Omenn GS, Goodman GE, Thornquist MD, Balmes J, Cullen MR, Glass A, Keogh JP, Meyskens FL, Valanis B, Williams JH, Barnhart S, Hammar S. 1996. Effects of a combination of beta carotene and vitamin A on lung cancer and cardiovascular disease. *New England Journal of Medicine* 334:1150–1155.

Oxman AD, Sackett DL, Guyatt GH. 1993. Users' guides to the medical literature. I. How to get started. The Evidence-Based Medicine Working Group. *Journal of the American Medical Association* 270:2093–2095.

Pauker SG. 1976. Coronary artery surgery: The use of decision analysis. *Annals of Internal Medicine* 85:8–18.

Pearl R. 1938. Tobacco smoking and longevity. *Science* 87:216–217.

People who drink as few as two soft drinks a week face nearly twice the risk of developing deadly cancer, study finds. 2010. *CBSNews Healthwatch*, February 9.

Petitti D. 2005. Triumphs in epidemiology. *Epidemiology Monitor* 26:1–3.

Pettenkofer M von. 1941. The value of health to a city: Two lectures delivered in 1873. *Bulletin of the History of Medicine* 10:473–503, 593–613.

Pinel, Philippe. 1807. Résultats d'observations et construction des tables pour servir à déterminer le degré de probabilité de la guérison des aliénés. *Mémoires de la classe des sciences mathématiques et physiques de l'Institut National de France,* Premier semestre: 169–205.

Poland GA, Poland CM, Howe CL. 2013. Influenza vaccine and Guillain-Barré syndrome: Making informed decisions. *Lancet* 381:1437–1439.

Politicians should not prescribe pills. 2010. *Financial Times*, July 14.

Porter D. 1999. *Health, Civilization, and the State: A History of Public Health from Ancient to Modern Times*. London: Routledge.

Porter R. 1997. *The Greatest Benefit to Mankind: A Medical History of Humanity*. London: Harper Collins.

Press DJ, Pharoah P. 2010. Risk factors for breast cancer: A reanalysis of two case-control studies from 1926 and 1931. *Epidemiology* 21:566–572.

Proctor RN. 1988. *Racial Hygiene: Medicine Under the Nazis*. Cambridge, MA: Harvard University Press.

Proctor RN. 2006. Angel H Roffo: The forgotten father of experimental tobacco carcinogenesis. *Bulletin of the World Health Organization* 84:494–496.

Proctor RN. 2012. *Golden Holocaust: Origins of the Cigarette Catastrophe and the Case for Abolition*. Berkeley: University of California Press.

Progestin: Hormone replacement therapy study halted. 2002. *CNN Health*, July 9.

Quetelet A. 1869. *Physique sociale: Essai sur le développement des facultés de l'homme*. Brussels: Issakoff.

Rabin RC. 2011. Fewer women dying of lung cancer. *New York Times*, April 12.

Ramsey GH. 1925. An epidemic of scarlet fever spread by ice cream. *American Journal of Hygiene* 5:669–681.

Researchers link deaths to social ills. 2011. *New York Times*, July 4.

Research shows extra calcium unnecessary. 2011. *West Australian*, May 25. http://au.news.yahoo.com/thewest/lifestyle/a/-/health/9513662/research-shows-extra-calcium-unnecessary/.

Riegelman RK. 2008. Undergraduate public health education: Past, present, and future. *American Journal of Preventive Medicine* 35:258–263.

Ringa V, Fritel X, Varnoux N, Zins M, Quelen C, Bouyer J. 2010. Discontinuation of hormone therapy in the French GAZEL cohort 1990–2006. *Fertility and Sterility* 94:1387–1391.

Risueño d'Amador B. 1837. *Mémoire sur le calcul des probabilités appliqué à la médecine*. Paris: Baillière.

Roe DA. 1973. *"A Plague of Corn": The Social History of Pellagra*. Ithaca, NY: Cornell University Press.

Roffo A. 1931. Durch Tabak beim Kaninchen entwickeltes Carcinom. *Zeitschrift fuer Krebsforshung* 33:321–332.

Rosborough TK, Bank CH, Cummings MK, Phillips PP, Pierach CA. 1990. MRFIT after 10.5 years. *Journal of the American Medical Association* 264:1534–1535.

Rose G. 1993. *The Strategy of Preventive Medicine*. New York: Oxford University Press.

Rose G, Day S. 1990. The population mean predicts the number of deviant individuals. *British Medical Journal* 301:1031–1034.

Rosen G. 1958. *A History of Public Health*. New York: MD Publications.

Rossouw JE, Anderson GL, Prentice RL, LaCroix AZ, Kooperberg C, Stefanick ML, Jackson RD, Beresford SA, Howard BV, Johnson KC, Kotchen JM, Ockene J. 2002. Risks and benefits of estrogen plus progestin in healthy postmenopausal women: Principal results from the Women's Health Initiative randomized controlled trial. *Journal of the American Medical Association* 288:321–333.

Rothman KJ. 1986. *Modern Epidemiology*. 1st ed. Boston: Little Brown.

Rusnock AA. 2002. *Vital Accounts: Quantifying Health and Population in Eighteenth-Century England and France*. Cambridge: Cambridge University Press

Sackett DL, Rosenberg WM, Gray JA, Haynes RB, Richardson WS. 1996. Evidence based medicine: What it is and what it isn't. *British Medical Journal* 312:71–72.

Salmon DA, Proschan M, Forshee R, Gargiullo P, Bleser W, Burwen DR, Cunningham F, Garman P, Greene SK, Lee GM, Vellozzi C, Yih WK, Gellin B, Lurie N. 2013. Association between Guillain-Barré syndrome and influenza A (H1N1) 2009 monovalent inactivated vaccines in the USA: A meta-analysis. *Lancet* 381:1461–1468.

Sanmuganathan PS, Ghahramani P, Jackson PR, Wallis EJ, Ramsay LE. 2001. Aspirin for primary prevention of coronary heart disease: Safety and absolute benefit related to coronary risk derived from meta-analysis of randomised trials. *Heart* 85:265–271.

Schairer E, Schoeniger E. 1943. Lungenkrebs und Tabakverbrauch. *Zeitschrift fuer Krebsforschung* 54:261–269.

Schairer E, Schoeniger E. 2001. Lung cancer and tobacco consumption. *International Journal of Epidemiology* 30:24–27.

Schroeder FH, Hugosson J, Roobol MJ, Tammela TL, Ciatto S, Nelen V, Kwiatkowski M, Lujan M, Lilja H, Zappa M, Denis LJ, Recker F, Berenguer A, Maattanen L, Bangma CH, Aus G, Villers A, Rebillard X, van der KT, Blijenberg BG, Moss SM, de Koning HJ, Auvinen A. 2009. Screening and prostate-cancer mortality in a randomized European study. *New England Journal of Medicine* 360:1320–1328.

Schwartz D, Flamant R, Lellouch J, Denoix PF. 1961. Results of a French survey on the role of tobacco, particularly inhalation, in different cancer sites. *Journal of the National Cancer Institute* 26:1085–1108.

Scientists identify genes for "extreme longevity." 2010. *AOL News*, July 1.

Shapiro S, Vennet W, Strax P, Venet L. 1988. *Periodic Screening for Breast Cancer: The Health Insurance Plan Project and Its Sequelae, 1963–1986*. Baltimore: Johns Hopkins University Press.

Sigerist HE. 1941. Introduction to Max von Pettenkofer, *"The Value of Health to a City": Two Lectures Delivered in 1873. Bulletin of the History of Medicine* 10:473–486.

Sigerist HE. 1951. *A History of Medicine*. Vol.1: *Primitive and Archaic Medicine*. New York: Oxford University Press.

Siler J, Garrison P, MacNeal W. 1914. Further studies of the Thompson–McFadden pellagra commission: A summary of the second progress report. *Journal of the American Medical Association* 63:1090–1093.

Sisson JC, Schoomaker EB, Ross JC. 1976. Clinical decision analysis: The hazard of using additional data. *Journal of the American Medical Association* 236:1259–1263.

Slack P. 1981. The disappearance of plague: An alternative view. *Economic History Review* 34:469–476.

Snow J. 1849. On the pathology and modes of communication of cholera. *London Medical Gazette* 44:745–752.

Snow J. 1855. *On the Mode of Communication of Cholera*. London: Churchill.

Soustelle J. 1955. *La vie quotidienne des Aztèques à la veille de la conquête espagnole*. Paris: Hachette.

Stampfer MJ. 2008. ITT for observational data: Worst of both worlds? *Epidemiology* 19 : 783–784, discussion 789–793.

Stephens T, Brynner R. 2001. *Dark Remedy: The Impact of Thalidomide and Its Revival as a Vital Medicine*. Cambridge, MA: Perseus.

Stocks P, Karn M. 1933. A co-operative study of the habits, home life, dietary and family histories of 450 cancer patients and of an equal number of control patients. *Annals of Eugenics* 5:237–279.

Stolley PD. 1991. When genius errs: R. A. Fisher and the lung cancer controversy. *American Journal of Epidemiology* 133:416–425.

Stone E. 1764. An account of the success of the bark of the willow in the cure of agues. *Philosophical Transactions* 53:195–200.

Study: Soda linked to pancreatic cancer. 2010. *CBS News*, February 9. http://www.cbsnews.com/stories/2010/02/09/health/main6189455.shtml.

Susser M, Stein Z. 2009. *Eras in Epidemiology*. New York: Oxford University Press.

Tehard B, Friedenreich CM, Oppert JM, Clavel-Chapelon F. 2006. Effect of physical activity on women at increased risk of breast cancer: Results from the E3N cohort study. *Cancer Epidemiology, Biomarkers, and Prevention* 15:57–64.

Terris M. 1964. *Golberger on Pellagra*. Baton Rouge: Louisiana State University Press.

Surgeon General's Advisory Committee. 1964. *Smoking and Health*. Public Health Service Publication no. 1103. Washington, DC: US Government Printing Office.

Therapeutic Trial Committee of the Medical Research Council. 1934. The serum treatment of lobar pneumonia: A report of the Therapeutic Trials Committee of the Medical Research Council. *British Medical Journal* 1:241–245.

Thomas RE, Jefferson T, Lasserson TJ. 2010. Influenza vaccination for healthcare workers who work with the elderly. *Cochrane Database Systematic Reviews* 2:CD005187.

Thompson I, Ankerst D, Chi C, Lucia M, Goodman P, Crowley J, Parnes H, Coltman C, Jr. 2005. Operating characteristics of prostate-specific antigen in men with an initial PSA level of 3.0 ng/mL or lower. *Journal of the American Medical Association* 294:66–71.

Troehler U. 2000. *To Improve the Evidence of Medicine: The 18th Century British Origins of a Critical Approach*. Edinburgh: Royal College of Physicians.

Troehler, U. 2008. James Lind and scurvy: 1747–1795. James Lind Library. http://www.jameslindlibrary.org/illustrating/articles/james-lind-and-scurvy-1747-to-1795. Accessed October 7, 2013.

Truswell AS, Hansen JDL. 1976. Medical research among the !Kung. In RB Lee and I De Vore, eds. *Kalahari Hunter-Gatherers*, 167–194. Cambridge, MA: Harvard University Press.

Vandenbroucke, JP. 2004. When are observational studies as credible as randomised trials? *Lancet* 363:1728–1731.

Vandenbroucke, JP. 2009. The HRT controversy: Observational studies and RCTs fall in line. *Lancet* 373:1233–1235.

Vandenbroucke J, Eelkman Rooda H, Beukers HM. 1991. Who made John Snow a hero? *American Journal of Epidemiology* 133:967–973.

Vandenbroucke JP, Pardoel VP. 1989. An autopsy of epidemiologic methods: The case of "poppers" in the early epidemic of the acquired immunodeficiency syndrome (AIDS). *American Journal of Epidemiology* 129:455–457.

Vitamins "lower risk of autism." 2011. *Sydney Morning Herald*, May 27. http://www.smh.com.au/lifestyle/wellbeing/vitamins-lower-risk-of-autism-20110526-1f6h8.html#ixzz1Nr3wccq3.

Volmink J. 2008. The willow as a Hottentot (Khoikhoi) remedy for rheumatic fever. *Journal of the Royal Society of Medicine* 101:321–323.

Walsh B. 2010. Cell phones and cancer: A study's muddled findings. *Time*, May 17. http://www.time.com/time/health/article/0,8599,1989740,00.html.

Wegwarth O, Schwartz LM, Woloshin S, Gaissmaier W, Gigerenzer G. 2012. Do physicians understand cancer screening statistics? A national survey of primary care physicians in the United States. *Annals of Internal Medicine* 156:340–349.

Weinberg W. 1913. *Die Kinder der Tuberkuloesen*. Leipzig: Hirzel.

Weindling P. 1989. *Health, Race, and German Politics Between National Unification and Nazism, 1870–1945*. New York: Cambridge University Press.

Weinstein M. 1980. *Clinical Decision Analysis*. Oxford: Saunders.

Wildner M, Hofman A. 2008. Re: Epidemiologic interactions, complexity, and the lonesome death of Max von Pettenkofer. *American Journal of Epidemiology* 168:119–120.

Wilhelm Weinberg. 2009. In *History of Epidemiology*. Updated February 26. http://www.epidemiology.ch/history/weinberg.htm.

Willett WC, Stampfer MJ, Manson JE, Colditz GA, Speizer FE, Rosner BA, Sampson LA, Hennekens CH. 1993. Intake of trans fatty acids and risk of coronary heart disease among women. *Lancet* 341:581–585.

Wilson R. 1966. *Feminine Forever*. New York: Evans.

Winkelstein W Jr. 2004. Vignettes of the history of epidemiology: Three firsts by Janet Elizabeth Lane-Claypon. *American Journal of Epidemiology* 160:97–101.

Wolfe ND, Dunavan CP, Diamond J. 2007. Origins of major human infectious diseases. *Nature* 447:279–283.

Wynder E, Graham E. 1950. Tobacco smoking as a possible etiologic factor in bronchiogenic carcinoma: A study of six hundred and eighty four proved cases. *Journal of the American Medical Association* 143:329–336.

Zinsser H. 1935. *Rats, Lice, and History*. Boston: Little, Brown.

# INDEX

Page numbers for endnotes include both chapter and endnote designation (e.g., 226n2:13 indicates page 226, chap. 2, note 13).